BACH FLOWER ESSENCES
AND
CHINESE MEDICINE

"In *Bach Flower Essences and Chinese Medicine* Pablo Noriega takes us into an exploration that has never been so thoroughly attempted: the intersection of Bach Flower Essence theory with that of Chinese Medicine. Both fields hold in high regard the role that the mind and emotions play in human health and suffering. Restoration of balance in the psycho-spiritual realm is highly prized by both paradigms. The brilliance of Bach's theory is in the careful observation of complex human conditions and the identification of plant energies that can harmonize dissonant mindsets. Chinese Medicine also prizes the study of the mind and emotions and how these relate to disease development and has carefully cataloged these in domains of human function known as the five organ systems. Noriega deftly weaves discussion of how these two systems inform one another, giving greater insight into both fields. He expands treatment options for practitioners of Chinese Medicine and broadens treatment context for practitioners of Flower Essence Therapy. This work will be of interest to all who enjoy traversing the boundaries between paradigms and who find satisfaction on the frontiers of intercultural exchange."

DAVID W. MILLER, M.D., FAAP, L.AC., DIPL. OM,
EAST-WEST INTEGRATED MEDICINE, LLC

BACH FLOWER ESSENCES

AND

CHINESE MEDICINE

PABLO NORIEGA

TRANSLATED BY LOEY COLEBECK

Healing Arts Press
Rochester, Vermont • Toronto, Canada

Healing Arts Press
One Park Street
Rochester, Vermont 05767
www.HealingArtsPress.com

Text stock is SFI certified

Healing Arts Press is a division of Inner Traditions International

Originally published in Spanish in 2012 under the title *Medicina China y Flores de Bach* by El Grano de Mostaza in Barcelona, Spain

First U.S. edition published in 2016 by Healing Arts Press

Note to the reader: *This book is intended as an informational guide. The remedies, approaches, and techniques described herein are meant to supplement, and not to be a substitute for, professional medical care or treatment. They should not be used to treat a serious ailment without prior consultation with a qualified health care professional.*

Library of Congress Cataloging-in-Publication Data

Names: Noriega, Pablo, 1962– | Colebeck, Loey, 1974– translator.

Title: Bach flower essences and Chinese medicine / Pablo Noriega ; translated by Loey Colebeck.

Other titles: Medicina China y flores de Bach. English | Flower essences and Chinese medicine

Description: First U.S. edition. | Rochester, Vermont : Healing Arts Press, [2016] | Originally published in Spanish in 2012 under the title: Medicina China y flores de Bach (Barcelona, Spain : by El Grano de Mostaza). | Includes bibliographical references and index.

Identifiers: LCCN 2015048236 (print) | LCCN 2016000111 (e-book) | ISBN 9781620555712 (pbk.) | ISBN 9781620555729 (e-book)

Subjects: LCSH: Flowers—Therapeutic use. | Homeopathy—Materia medica and therapeutics. | Naturopathy. | Medicine, Chinese.

Classification: LCC RX615.F55 N6713 2016 (print) | LCC RX615.F55 (e-book) | DDC 615.5/32—dc23

LC record available at http://lccn.loc.gov/2015048236

Printed and bound in the United States by Lake Book Manufacturing, Inc.

The text stock is SFI certified. The Sustainable Forestry Initiative. program promotes sustainable forest management.

10 9 8 7 6 5 4 3 2 1

Text design and layout by Priscilla Baker

This book was typeset in Garamond Premier Pro with Brioso Pro, Shelley Script, and Avant Garde used as display typefaces

To send correspondence to the author of this book, mail a first-class letter to the author c/o Inner Traditions • Bear & Company, One Park Street, Rochester, VT 05767, and we will forward the communication, or contact the translator directly at **www.Mindisbodytherapies.com.**

Contents

Part 1
An Introduction to
Chinese Medicine

Translator's Foreword

*I*f you ask any resident of Barcelona if they know about the Bach Flowers, *las Flores de Bach,* chances are better than not that the answer is yes. There is more than one school in that city dedicated exclusively to the study of Flower Essence Therapy (*terapia floral*) and many other schools of complementary or traditional medicine that offer serious coursework in the Bach Remedies alongside acupuncture, osteopathy, naturopathy, and so on. Some pharmacies mix personalized Flower Essence formulas. Several regional and national associations of Flower Essence Therapy publish bulletins, organize conferences, and provide professional support to practitioners, among other activities. One of them, SEDIBAC (Societat per l'Estudi I Difusió de la Teràpia del Dr. Bach de Catalunya, or the Catalonia Society for the Study and Diffusion of Dr. Bach's Therapy), hosts weekly meetings with in-depth study of the Flowers and related areas. This is the context in which I had the great fortune to meet Pablo Noriega.

The situation is similar in many parts of Latin America. Cuba introduced Bach Flower Therapy into its health-care system, Nicaragua has officially recognized Flower Essence Therapy, Chile sees wide diffusion and outreach practice, and international conferences in the field are held in Mexico. The list goes on. There are more books published about Flower Essence Therapy in Spanish than in any other language.

I hope this to be one of many forthcoming translations bringing

Flower Essence Therapy as a serious clinical practice back to the English-speaking world, where it originated. My heart-felt gratitude to all those who are participating in its development.

LOEY COLEBECK
MINNEAPOLIS, APRIL 2015

Loey (Loyola) Colebeck is an accredited Flower Essence Therapist through SEDIBAC. She trained at various institutions in Barcelona where she lived for eleven years, working with women in movement therapy. She has published articles and lectured at SEDIBAC's fourth biennial Flower Therapy conference in 2013. She currently teaches and practices clinical Flower Essence Therapy in Minneapolis.

Foreword

*I*f I were more cynical, the feeling I'd be having about the arrival of this book would be relief. "What's the name of Pablo's book?" "There's no book relating Chinese Medicine with the Bach Flower Remedies?" "When is Pablo's book coming out?" These and other similar questions from students, colleagues, and patients have been chasing me daily for years, with recalcitrant continuity. There exists just one person, Pablo Noriega himself, who has probably suffered all this and much more. And worse yet, all I could do was to insist time and again, especially when he'd come to Barcelona, the need for him to write the glorious book, almost like a family member or friend who pressures the alcoholic or drug addict to go into treatment. Why couldn't he publish the material that he'd repeatedly given in his courses?

But now, reading the manuscript, I understand perfectly why it is that a work like this cannot be precipitated. One who is connected with wise Oriental philosophy, as is the author, knows the value of not rushing phases and the advisability of being accountable.

I do not believe that I am influenced by either the quality of his humanity or the friendship that ties me to Pablo when I say that this book is magnificent.

First, because the person who wrote it knows exactly what he's talking about. Despite his modesty, he knows very well both of the disciplines he covers. Second, because it's not a rough approximation, as he says it is, but a knowledgeable integration of Chinese Medicine and Bach Flower Therapy.

The introduction is absolutely illuminating. The in-depth look at each organ from the perspective of Chinese Medicine is brilliant. But the most interesting part is that the Flowers aren't forcefully shoved in at the end of the book in an isolated and shy appendix, but instead they show their faces continuously throughout the book, confirming, once again, Pablo's depth of knowledge.

The individual tale of each Flower viewed from Chinese Medicine is totally expository and profound.

Finally, the navigation charts strike me as surprisingly delicious and useful. A true guide for us land sailors who aspire to navigate the choppy waters of signs, symptoms, emotions, and thoughts—in short, the sea of knowledge.

DR. RICARDO OROZCO
BARCELONA, JANUARY 2012

Dr. Orozco is a licensed physician and has been a Bach Flower Therapist since 1984. He cofounded SEDIBAC (Catalonia Society for the Study and Diffusion of Dr. Bach's Therapy) in 1993 and has been training Bach Flower Therapists since 1994. He is the founder of Institut Anthemon (Anthemon Institute) in Barcelona where over two thousand Flower Therapists have been trained. He is widely recognized for his conception of the Transpersonal Patterns of the Bach Flowers, is the author and coauthor of several books, and gives courses in various countries.

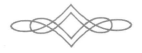

Bridging Chinese Medicine and Bach Flower Therapy

*P*aths are made by walking, the beloved Spanish poet Antonio Machado once said.

And likewise, the paths lead us, against all previsions, up to unimaginable heights and down to the deepest depths, without consulting us in the least.

They change direction, and maps do very little to help us.

In this book, I wish to share with the reader those paths along which I was, more often than not, taken. And, naïveté aside, I accept that I also consented to follow them with joy, though not exempt of darkness.

Chinese Medicine is an art, and not of the simplest kind. It has a structure that has been built on centuries of clinical practice, firmly supported by a theoretical body that sinks its roots into the heart of Chinese culture.

To incorporate other knowledge is, to say the least, risky business.

Knowing that barbaric peoples who took up the task of conquering China invariably ended up being assimilated into its culture, and thus knocking down the dream of forging a nation in its image and likeness, we will try, on the one hand, to bring the marvelous and subtle efficacy of Flower Essences a little closer to Chinese Medicine, and, on the other, to offer Flower Essence Therapy sips from the endless, crystal spring of the wisdom of Chinese Medicine.

Supporting Flower Essence Therapy with knowledge from Chinese

Medicine opens up a very wide range of possibilities, some of them already explored, and this book draws together points of reference from which I've been working, with the goal of stimulating thought and orienting clinical practice.

I know that many colleagues practice Chinese Medicine and use Flower Essences, and that many others, trained in the field of Flower Essence Therapy, nourish themselves from concepts and diagnostic possibilities of Chinese Medicine. So another goal of this book is to propose a dialogue, a place where we can meet to enrich each other and construct the bridge together.

As a Flower Essence Therapist, I have found myself in various situations with patients who found it quite complicated to talk about their emotions, or to even give a hint of a sentiment, while on the other hand talking about their physical suffering didn't pose any difficulty. So I began using the relationships that for centuries Chinese Medicine has been establishing between emotions and physical complaints, and this allowed me to see which emotions, sentiments, and Psyches or psychospiritual aspects were at play.

In observing imbalances in the Blood, Energy, and body fluids, Chinese Medicine includes disturbances that these imbalances generate in the emotions and the Psyches.

That which lies beneath physiological, emotional, psychological, and mental processes is Energy. Its equilibrium, in quantity and quality, depends upon factors as delicate as one's own attitude and the opportunities available for developing one's abilities.

With this book, it is my intention to: bring the Flower Essence Therapist closer to knowledge from Chinese Medicine that could be useful, contribute guidelines for diagnosis, treatment and strategies, and shine a light on a side of Flower Essences that until now has not been revealed.

The Flowers undoubtedly have many facets yet unseen that will reveal themselves as Flower Essence Therapy itself evolves and through contributions from other disciplines.

I occasionally reflect using basic concepts from Chinese Medicine as a point of departure, taking advantage of its symbolic richness; the ideas I've formulated respond to my own experience, both theoretical and practical, and I propose their application and their debate.

Practitioners of Chinese Medicine will find suggestions for using the Flowers within the framework of their knowledge, allowing them to incorporate the Flowers in their practice, to establish relationships, and to approach (among other possibilities) the regulation of emotions and Spirit—factors that, if not taken into consideration, lay many treatments out cold.

I am currently working on relationships that offer the Chinese Medicine practitioner more possibilities. Nevertheless it seemed appropriate to begin with a book that would bring some of Chinese Medicine's knowledge regarding the world of the psyche closer to the Flower Essence Therapist.

This book does not contain everything. We know that is impossible. This book necessarily leaves empty spaces and doubts so that the bridge, or whatever each person wishes to call it, remains under construction and so that these doubts lead to other books, other authors, other places, including other bridges beyond the Flowers and Chinese Medicine.

For some people it may be a bridge to . . . entirely unknown places.

What is being proposed in this book is not "the truth" about Chinese Medicine and the Bach Flower Remedies. Instead, I feel it to be a beginning, although it speaks of things that started long before I was born. It's a look at how this two-way bridge may be constructed and traveled, and it is open to continuous construction, to demolition and reconstruction with other materials from other subject matter—or it might end right here where it started. All this to say, may it follow its destiny.

As if it were a boat, we launch it into the river of knowledge that has been flowing for millennia. Whether it floats and whether it sails will be seen.

What is clear is that what I offer comes from the generosity of my teachers who had the enormous goodness and patience to transmit to me that which they themselves received and for which I am profoundly grateful. Especially to Ricardo Orozco, with his tenacity, enormous friendship, and conception of the Transpersonal Patterns,* not only has

---

*[Transpersonal Patterns, developed by Dr. Ricardo Orozco in his handbook about topical applications of the Bach Flower Remedies, *Flores de Bach: Manual para Aplicaciones Locales,* opened the gates for investigating new uses of the Remedies and are referred to, oftentimes implicitly, throughout the text of this book. —*Trans.*]

he witnessed the birth of this book but was also one of its most power-ful driving forces.

As the painter Roberto Bosco, one of my teachers, says, "We are a link in the chain. With luck, a word in the book."

If it is meant to be, so be it.

Acknowledgments

From the roots, we form ourselves out of many others.
Light is borrowed, the body an instant.

The web that unites us is limitless.

A sparkle suddenly vibrates in the air. Someone believes it was he who gave it life, that he was the one who mixed the blues and the ivies, the looks, the liquors, the delicate leaves that never touch the ground, and the water of the night.

Someone laughs, seated, soaking his feet in the liquid tide of life, someone who knows that the web is infinite, that the roots are interlaced, that we are made of Earth and Sky, that the sparkle of one was forged with tiny filings from the light of everyone.

I offer my gratitude to Guillermo Stilstein, who very early on showed us the door to Chinese Medicine and Tai Chi and with whom a long road has been traveled, one I hope to continue walking together.

Many thanks to Dr. Diana Carballo, who accepted my enthusiasm and guided me through my many questions, and an enormous hug for Héctor Carballo and for Diana and Héctor's mom, Fanny T. Socolovsky: may my hugs reach them in whichever place of infinity they find themselves.

Thank you to Dr. Tze Ching Hsiang, with whom I continued studying acupuncture and Chinese Medicine. Through his work with me, theory began to unfold and to flow into my practice.

My gratitude and warmth to one of my teachers and friends, Ricardo

"El chino" Fernández Herrero, who taught me in class, during lunch, in practice, while sipping yerba maté. He shared with me his nutritional method and deep knowledge in many areas of Chinese Medicine, as well as moments of relaxed friendship during long stretches of our lives.

Dr. He Yi Ming, through his practice and humility, taught me without me being particularly conscious of it. One of his ways was helping me maintain health with Chinese herbs.

Around this same time, another great teacher, the painter Roberto Bosco, passing on that which his own teacher, Demetrio Urruchúa, had passed to him—painting and drawing, but much more than that, a way of seeing the world very close to Daoism. To him and to his family, the painter Zulma Gallardo, Cristina y Romina. A word of gratitude as well to a friend from that period, the painter Alejandro Parisi.

To Dr. Gabriel Carrascosa Solar, companion and friend, with whom I share and learn much. Thank you.

To Dr. Ana María Soerensen and Dr. Edgardo Soerensen, for the training I received from them, enormously generous, disinterested and humble. It signified a transcendental 180-degree turn in my way of looking at medicine. Their contribution to natural medicine, to biological medicine, is incalculable. They have trained and continue to train many people.

My gratitude for the teachings of Bárbara Espeche, in whose institution I studied Flower Essence Therapy.

To Eduardo Grecco: thanks to him I was able to begin to share the first steps of this work and to access a very valuable Chinese Medicine library. My first trips to Mexico and Barcelona were arranged with his help.

Big thanks to my grandfather, Dr. Tomás Argentino Ortíz Luna, greatness, humility and kindness, another one from whom I learned without realizing it.

To my uncle Dr. Tomás Alejandro Ortíz Luna, whose path within the medical system shows, in practice, how integration can look.

Many thanks to my friend Dr. Ramiro Velazco, investigator and great practitioner of forms of traditional medicine. Innovator. He taught me in consultation and during long hours of sharing his knowledge with me.

To Dr. Alfonso Masi Elizalde, homeopath, who showed me in

action and over the course of three days how an ailment of many years can be cured.

To Dr. Eduardo Yahbes, homeopath. His work with me led me to another therapeutic practice.

My gratitude to Susana Fryc, director of Instituto Sadhana (Sadhana Institute) in Buenos Aires, where my work has been able to unfold with total liberty and support.

To Claudia Stern, director of Cefyn, in Buenos Aires. Thanks to her I was able to begin and to continue to share this material in that city.

To my student-colleagues at Cefyn: the work with them is intense; it's pure impulse and affection. Thank you.

To my student-colleagues at Instituto Sadhana, more joyous and affectionate learning and sharing.

All of them are building the bridge between Chinese Medicine and the Bach Flowers.

Many thanks to Lourdes Campos and María Julia Falcón of the Instituto de Terapeutas Florales Mount Vernon (Mount Vernon Institute of Flower Essence Therapists) of Santiago, Chile. Their disinterested work in supporting and spreading Flower Essence Therapy, along with the work for and with the people there, is immense and very valuable.

Thank you to those in Chile: colleagues, students, and patients. To my colleagues Carolina Sougarret and Gonzalo Valdés for their work and enthusiasm, and to Ronny Cornejo.

Many thanks to my friends and colleagues of the "Foursome" Seminar in Barcelona: Ricardo Orozco, Jordi Cañellas, and Josep Guarch. And the other bald guy in Cuba, honorary member of the pentibaldies, Boris Rodriguez. You are my brothers.

Jordi Cañellas and I share the joy of getting together and talking about the Flowers and medicine, and somehow magical doors seem to open. Thanks, also, to his wife, Marga, and their lovely children.

Josep Guarch, soul brother, deep, a great therapist and astrologer, with whom many good times have been shared in Barcelona and Buenos Aires. Thanks as well to Leire, Pau, and Maialen for sharing and for receiving me in their home in Barcelona.

Boris Rodriguez, clinical psychologist, defender of the scientific recognition of Bach Flower Remedies.

A very many great thanks to Ricardo Orozco, for his enormous work with the Bach Flower Remedies, his contribution of the Transpersonal Patterns, thanks to which I was able to begin putting together pieces of the bridge between Chinese Medicine and the Bach Flowers, as have many other people in other disciplines. An inexhaustible trainer of Flower Essence Therapists and a great and beloved friend. He pushed my work forward in many ways. The possibility of sharing it and developing it is due to his unconditional support during these ten years. And thanks to Pilar, who along with Ricardo receive me in their home when I'm in Barcelona.

Much gratitude to Institut Anthemon (Anthemon Institute), of which I form part, and where I've been developing, thanks to Ricardo Orozco, work that has been going on for ten years now.

I wish to express my deep gratitude to the SEDIBAC (Societat per l'Estudi I Difusió de la Teràpia del Dr. Bach de Catalunya, or the Catalonia Society for the Study and Diffusion of Dr. Bach's Therapy), where I've so often been invited to give workshops and seminars.

Thank you to the Institut Homeopatic de Catalunya (Homeopathic Institute of Catalonia), for the work I did there.

Thank you to Gabriel Nieto, director of the Escuela Taoísta del Sur (South Daoist School). His work changed my view of medicine and Daoist practices and inspired me to change. Thanks to Eduardo Alexander, professor of Daoist arts, investigator who developed the excellent thesis that I mention repeatedly throughout this book. Gabriel and Eduardo have both generously shared with me and with many others the fruit of their work.

My gratitude to Walter Pampin and Paula Betti, friends and companions in Daoist practice. Their affection, wisdom, and generosity arrived during both difficult times and in the simplest and most peaceful of times too.

Thank you to my very dear Francesc Mariegas. It's true that we seem to be twins in so many things. Thank you for your friendship and kindness, for the long talks in Barcelona, Buenos Aires and Uruguay, about Daoism, Chinese Medicine, and the thousands of topics that fascinate us, for your book *El Tao del Cambio* (The Dao of Change). Kisses and thanks to your family, to Dinorah, and to wonderful little Irenita.

Thank you to María E. Ortíz Luna and Rodolfo Noriega, my parents.

To Nélida Mir, another mother. To Oscar Massa, where my gratitude may find him, another father. To Jorge Domínguez, yet another father.

And for Andrea Rur, my wife and colleague, companion of a long path. Enormous thanks for the love, the transformation, life, and, of course, for working so much on this book and on the material of innumerable seminars over the course of all these years.

Very special thanks to my son, Lautaro Noriega, light, energy, and talent, for all the help and for the time that I spent writing and working instead of playing.

A heart-felt thank you to everyone.
Thank you to the whole of everything.
Thank you.

INTRODUCTION

Chinese Medicine
and Bach Flower Therapy

*T*raditional Chinese Medicine as we know it today is the sum of knowledge and practices that has been forged over the course of thousands of years.

What some authors call Classical Chinese Medicine was developed in China during some sixteen centuries. After this period, the expansive influence of Western culture began to mark the decline of this way of conceiving Chinese Medicine.

In 1927, it was prohibited and considered by the political powers to be a load of superstition, and after the Communist Revolution it was reborn under the name of Traditional Chinese Medicine, constituting a synthesis of traditional culture with modern science and concepts.

This process excluded, and gave a different meaning to, fundamental knowledge from Classical Chinese Medicine, as it was considered mystical in nature.

Everything stated up to this point is not meant in any way to detract from Traditional Chinese Medicine and its merits, nor deny China's historical and political necessity with respect to the management of its medicine. Nevertheless, it is in Classical Chinese Medicine where we find a communion of ideas and practices corresponding with Dr. Bach's postulates.*

---

*[For beginning reading on the postulates of Dr. Edward Bach (1886–1936), see his book *Heal Thyself. —Trans.*]

1

Following the work of Eduardo Alexander ("Nutrindo a vitalidade"), three levels of knowledge and practices may be recognized in Classical Chinese Medicine: the Celestial Level, the Human Level, and the Earthly Level.

From the viewpoint of the Celestial Level, illness comes about as a consequence of ignoring one's internal nature, of not heeding one's divine calling or "mandate of Heaven," and of not using one's abilities bestowed as a means for manifesting in the world that for which one is destined. A disconnection is generated between one's being and the primordial source of vitality.

It is important, then, to favor self-knowledge and the development of each being's own potential in harmony with society. As Alexander says, "Indefinitely sustaining the development of vital energy" is also sought. Practices geared toward achieving immortality pertain to this level.

At the Human Level, illness is a product of becoming fixed in one form of perceiving and processing the world, which determines one's constitution and thus provokes excesses, deficiencies, and disorders in the circulation of Energy in varying systems. Other factors on the Human Level that create illness are:

- Disturbances that arise when a person fails to adapt his or her activities to the particular energetic qualities of each season
- Loss of mental stillness and emotional harmony
- Erosion of Essence,* generally as a consequence of sexual activity

Cultivating the Virtues, as explained in chapter 6 on the Psyches, is considered to be a therapeutic practice that helps one reconnect with the process of discovering one's internal nature and also favors the dissolution of the constitutional binding. Regulating and balancing the above-mentioned aspects is also sought in order to minimize their incidence as factors generating disturbances, as these disturbances block the cultivation of the Virtues and thus a return to a full state of health. Therapy at this level is also geared toward prevention and longevity.

At the Earthly Level, some factors that create illness are climatic

---

*[Essence is explained in chapter 4, "Energy and Blood." —*Trans.*]

(such as wind, the cold of winter, the heat of summer, dampness, fire, and dryness) along with emotions, epidemics, inadequate nutrition, and sexual excesses, among others. At this level, therapeutic practice is oriented toward curing illnesses, eliminating pathological factors that create illness, and harmonizing imbalances. Health has already deteriorated and must be reestablished. Emotions have become a factor in illness here and must be regulated so they do not affect the Organs with which they are closely related and do not disturb the circulation of Blood and Energy. At the Human Level, on the other hand, harmonizing emotions is sought so that they do not become factors generating illness (prevention is the therapeutic practice at this level) and especially to avoid disturbing the serenity of the conscious mind.

Having assumed that Emotions, as factors in imbalances, are present at all three levels, we can now begin to discern some of the Flowers' possible effects and also appreciate that Dr. Bach's postulates are very much aligned with the concept of illness in Classical Chinese Medicine.

The Flowers also offer a way to cultivate the Virtues that far exceeds intellectual attempts and good intentions; many times these attempts alone are unable to touch that which is essential—that which is truly intimate and authentic—in the way the Flowers are able to do by permeating the connection with source.

Drawing from Dr. Bach's postulates, we know that the Flower Remedies help draw out our internal nature, within social and cultural conventions, and unlock our potential so we can exercise them in the context of the soul's mandate. This is to say, the Flowers help us attain our destiny in harmony with the times and the society in which we live.

In Bach's own words, "We each have a divine mission in this world, and our souls use our minds and bodies as instruments to do this work" (*Collected Writings of Edward Bach,* chapter 2, "Free Thyself"). He further said "that certain Herbs, by bringing us solace, bring us closer to our Divinity" (*Collected Writings,* part 2, "Second Masonic Conference").

Notice how much this resembles the therapeutic orientation at the Celestial and Human Levels in Classical Chinese Medicine.

And so you can see how the concepts developed and explored throughout this book may help us understand different aspects of Chinese Medicine.

Part 1

An Introduction to Chinese Medicine

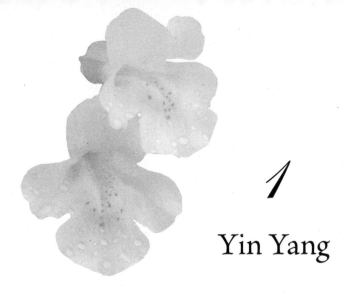

1

Yin Yang

hese two words no longer sound strange to us. Their diffusion in the West has been astounding, even to the point of being used to brand various products. Along with the modern Tai Chi symbol (☯), yin and yang have spread throughout the West, and there are probably more people who have heard these words than those who haven't.

This mass diffusion is quite new. In ancient times, knowledge that allowed access to wisdom and traditional sciences was transmitted to just a few people or groups and in a rather restricted manner. Large-scale diffusion of knowledge necessarily simplifies its contents, so with that in mind, let's dedicate some time to get to know more about this exciting view of the universe.

The sages of ancient times, like Laozi and Zhuang Zhu, tell us of the impenetrable origin of the universe: Dao. They revealed to us that it is a unity of two aspects.

One aspect transcends, unmanifest, that of nonbeing, the origin of all things that also sustains and nourishes all things. It is the primordial void, mentioned in texts as *Wuji,* out of which the manifest world is generated. This is a state of nondifferentiation in which original universal Energy is full and complete, with no distinction between one thing and another, with no thing having emerged as an individual separate from unity.

The other aspect is imminent, manifest, the multiplicity of things. It is said that it arises after the birth of Heaven and Earth.

We must remember that even though we are talking about them separately, these two facets form part of a unity. The Dao transcends this explicatory duality.

In the process of manifestation, Energy takes on two differentiated aspects, yin and yang. Yang is the active pole, and yin is the static pole. Form and shape are produced out of the interaction of these two poles.

The ancient sages drew on yin and yang to describe the nature of things and the changes of Heaven and Earth. This conception of the universe is the root and base of all the traditional Chinese sciences from art to engineering.

Like in other areas of knowledge in China, yin and yang build a fundamental pillar in the practice of medicine, both in theory and practice.

Yin and yang were linked to the Sun and the Moon and their characteristics. Their meaning naturally expanded until it applied to the shadow side and the sunny side of a mountain. They could literally be translated as shadow and light, respectively, or better yet, light and no light. In written Chinese, the character that corresponds to yin refers to that side of a mountain or hill that does not receive light, and the character corresponding to yang describes the side that is illuminated.

Going upon what the characters reveal to us about yin and yang, we can begin to understand which sorts of things could be attributed to yin and which others to yang. Try to evoke the feeling and appearance of a shadowed side of a hill. It is darker, cooler, less shiny, and the eyes can rest a bit, less damaged by brightness.

On the other hand, on the side with full sun, everything is in plain view and details that are difficult to see in the shadow are visible here. More Heat can be felt and everything tends to be more active.

Continuing with the characters, they both, in part, mean "hill, mound, or mountain." The character related to yang also shows us the Sun sending its rays of light from the horizon, denoting activity, Movement, Heat, projection. The character related to yin, along with the part representing "mountain," includes the characters "now and clouds." These two words refer to a moment in which there is less light as a cloud places itself between the Sun and Earth. The cloud also carries water, Dampness. The load that the cloud carries is heavier than the pure light of the Sun's rays.

We have been mentioning some attributes related to what the

characters for yin and yang insinuate; the notions of a sunny side and shadowed side of a mountain help us to deduce these attributes. So, that which is related to Heat, light, daytime, activity, and lightness are manifestations of the yang condition. Cold, dark, night, stillness, and heaviness are expressions of the yin condition.

With this, we begin to have some parameters for classifying objects and phenomena according to the yin-yang criteria, just as they were viewed in the classical texts of Chinese culture, and, of course, in the most important Chinese Medicine texts.

Nothing escapes classification in yin and yang. In the manifest world, we find in every object or phenomenon a "sunny" or "cloudy" aspect—the two opposing sides whose emblematic representatives are yin and yang. These opposing aspects are in conflict but are also interdependent.

Yin yang invites us to notice a union of opposites, which certainly modifies the usual Western point of view where opposites would not appear to have any relationship with each other, as if they were two separate things.

Out of unity, duality arises. We can, then, view duality as something that reminds us of unity and carries us toward unity. This becomes a less arduous task when we understand that opposites are not disconnected, that they are mutually influential, and that together they generate the development of events, complete each other, and explain each other.

Since ancient times, yin and yang were used to understand and explain changes in nature. Continuous transformation, or change, is, as it's been said many times, the only constant. If we think in terms of absolute and relative, Movement, growth, and decline are absolute; they are permanently happening. Immobility and balance are relative.

The *Huang Di Nei Jing* says "Yin Yang is a universal law, the key for analyzing and synthesizing the many objective things, the source of all change and the internal grounds for birth, evolution and extinction. Despite the existence of endless secrets in the world, they are without exception born of Yin and Yang. Thus, diagnosis and treatment of illness must be based on the essential problem of Yin and Yang" (Lu, *A Complete Translation of The Yellow Emperor's Classic of Internal Medicine and the Difficult Classic*).

TABLE 1.1. SOME YIN-YANG RELATIONSHIPS

Yin	Yang
Darkness	Light
Moon	Sun
Square	Circle
Space	Time
North	South
West	East
Right	Left
Shadow	Clarity
Cold	Heat
Internal	External
Matter	Energy
Substantial	Insubstantial
Tangible	Intangible
Contraction	Expansion
Depression	Excitement
Stillness	Movement
Rest	Activity
Water	Fire
Body	Spirit
Feminine	Masculine
Receive	Emit
Internal genitals	External genitals
Night	Day
Below	Above
Dampness	Dryness
Emptiness	Fullness
Hypersomnia	Insomnia
Lack of appetite	Appetite
Hypothermia	Fever
Chronic illnesses	Acute illnesses
Congestion	Inflammation
Heavy	Light

Ever-Present Yin and Yang

Once something comes to be in the manifest world, yin and yang are always there. No matter what it is that we may be looking at, considering in theory, or perceiving in any of the ways that humans can perceive, we are in the presence of these two aspects.

If we are able to take this constant into account, we will be capable of contacting both sides of any situation from a perspective of the whole. It is habitual to perceive only one aspect of a thing or a situation, leaving us ignorant about inherent cycles and alternation.

Alternation of opposites generates permanent Movement, which is what makes everything change. No phenomenon exists absolutely, on its own but rather is made comprehensible and exists thanks to its comparison with its opposite, the relationship between these two opposites. It is common knowledge, but let's repeat it anyway: we know when it is cold because we've experienced heat; relaxation makes sense thanks to the existence of tension; and life takes on meaning because death is there showing us the other side of the coin. That is how our perception works and everything can be observed from the perspective of yin yang, revealing the two aspects of each thing, situation, phenomenon, Movement, person, expression.

Yin Yang into Infinity

It is interesting to note also that, as well as each thing having two aspects, yin yang also exists within each aspect. If we take yin as the point of reference, we see that we can also divide it into yin yang, over and over, into infinity. The following examples will help to better explain this point. In full summer, the intensity of the Sun's heat melts our very thoughts, but nevertheless, under the lush canopy of a tree, protected on the side of a hill that casts a refreshing shadow, there is a cool puddle. Here in summer, which corresponds to yang, we find water, below a tree, a refuge of yin. In other words, yin within yang. The inverse: it is so cold outside that one could easily be frozen solid, but indoors, in the kitchen, the oven is lit, radiating such a balmy warmth that one must remove outer layers of clothing. Yang within yin.

Winter corresponds to yin. Daytime in winter corresponds to yang within yin; nighttime in winter is yin within yin.

One day in class, we allowed ourselves the pleasure of viewing a beautiful painting by Marc Chagall from the viewpoint of yin and yang, and among the things we noticed we saw that, as if asking for forgiveness, various interlaced shadows appeared in the most luminous areas of the painting. These shadows clearly highlighted the luminosity of the light. Yin within yang.

Relationships between Yin and Yang

Opposition and Mutual Restriction

Each pair of opposites, even the ones that we appreciate almost unconsciously, are represented by yin yang.

The world has within itself two sides, two opposing and complementary faces. As it's been said, everything under the Sun has a dark side and a light side.

It is important to keep in mind that this opposition is relative and by no means absolute. In order to determine that some aspect corresponds to yin, for example, we need the other piece for comparison. The table, compared to the floor, is higher. So we would say that it is more yang than the floor. But the same table compared to the ceiling corresponds to yin, leaving yang to correspond to the ceiling.

Something else is important to mention. We have just used high-low as the pair of opposites for comparing ceiling to table and table to floor. But if, on the other hand, we used light-shadow, and we saw that the table was more illuminated than the ceiling, we would have to say that the table is more yang than the ceiling.

So we see that yin and yang are not intrinsic qualities of things. When we catalog something as yin or yang, it is vitally important to know what we are comparing it to; which pairs or opposites we choose to compare will determine whether something is relatively yin or yang.

Yin and yang oppose each other while also forming a unit. They are complementary opposites. As opposites they limit each other, and paradoxically, this confrontation is what creates balance. Thanks to yin's opposition to the excess growth of yang, and vice versa, wholeness is maintained. We see this opposition in the mutual limitation of growth and decline. When one aspect grows, the other is reduced. When yang grows, yin decreases, and the reverse is also true. What is more, this push and pull happens cyclically, each aspect growing or declining in turn.

If yin diminishes, yang doesn't miss the opportunity to grow, and vice versa. Each measure of change is disputed in a way that is balanced and equal.

We are talking about balance, but as we hinted earlier, it is about a dynamic and cyclical balance, and this can be appreciated in the classic example of the progression of the seasons. As it becomes colder and winter draws closer, heat diminishes, and we get further away from summer. As heat increases and cold diminishes, we are headed toward summer. Because this alternation is cyclical, the seasons happen one after the other. Seen this way, the cycle or movement of the seasons is circular, and it isn't so simple to say, for example, whether summer is behind us or ahead of us. This cyclical concept of time marks a fundamental difference with the concept of time in the West. The passing of time is circular, so it isn't all that important to set out on a straight line toward a goal but rather to follow a circular path that rises and falls and to continue, to remain steady. The alternation of yin and yang induces the cycle.

When the relative balance resulting from the mutual opposition and limitation of yin yang is lost, illness ensues. One aspect is exaggerated and the other is deficient. A typical example: a person with high fever (excess yang) and with dry, wrinkly skin and thirst (decreased yin).

Interdependence

We now know about the intimate relationships between yin and yang, and it won't surprise us that one cannot exist without the other. Opposites exist together at once, the old "two sides of the coin." So without below, above becomes nonsense; without night, forget about day. If one of the aspects ceases to exist, the other disappears or loses its original meaning.

Continuing with the concept of interdependence, excitation instigates the inhibition to reveal oneself. Inhibition creates excitation.

In the *Tao Te Ching* (Levi, *The Complete Tao Te Ching*), Laozi expresses:

It is because everyone recognizes
beauty as beauty that there is ugliness.
It is because everyone knows
what is good that there is bad.
Being and Nonbeing engender one another,
difficult and easy complete each other,
long and short give each other form,
high and low complement each other,
sound and silence harmonize each other,
before and after succeed each other,
that is the law of nature.

Let's continue with some more traditional examples. We couldn't speak of circulation without Blood. Circulation is a functional aspect—yang—and Blood is matter in fluid form—yin. However, how could Blood circulate (fluid in movement, a manifestation of yang), without arteries (a yin aspect in this case), which limits the movement of Blood to a precise path?

It is in this way that Blood can fulfill its purpose. In order to carry out one of the two aspects, the other must also be taken into account.

Xie Zhufan and Liao Jiazhen in *Traditional Chinese Internal Medicine*, say:

The interdependence of *yin* and *yang* is also used to represent pathological changes. Since *yin* and *yang* rely on each other for existence, impairment of *yin* impedes the generation of *yang*; impairment of *yang* impedes the generation of *yin*. For example, persistent impairment of the digestive function may lead to malnutrition and anemia—deficiency of *yin* caused by impairment of *yang*. Acute massive Blood loss may give rise to failure of peripheral circulation—impairment of *yang* due to deficiency of *yin*.

Growth and Decline

Through their growth and decline, yin and yang maintain a dynamic balance. Alternating periods of growth and decline is a manifestation, as we've already stated, of the opposition and mutual limitation between yin and yang.

To maintain equilibrium, yin and yang are continuously making adjustments between themselves, and if their equilibrium is lost, they change their proportions in order to come back into harmony. The alternation of yin's or yang's predominance, in growth and decline, is of vital importance for the body's functioning. When an uncompensated imbalance occurs, disorders ensue.

There are four ways in which yin and yang express their imbalances:

- There is much yang. *Excess yang brings about a reduction of yin, consuming and debilitating it.*
- There is much yin. *Excess yin generates a reduction of yang.*
- There is little yang. *When yang is deficient, yin is in relative excess.*
- There is little yin. *When yin is deficient, yang is in relative excess.*

Let's look at this a little more closely. When yang is in excess, yin is diminished, but the principal imbalance is "excess yang," which creates a reduction of yin as a consequence.

When there is a yin deficiency, yang appears to be in excess, but only relative to the yin deficiency, which is the primary factor and whose consequence is a slightly "false" predominance of yang.

The same is true for excess yin and for yang deficiency.

If we wanted to use a fruity metaphor, not totally exact but still helpful, we might say the following: see this crate of pretty green apples and red apples in equal amounts? Well, let's add thirty red apples. Now the proportion is off; there is an excess of red apples. Likewise, if we had added thirty green apples, we would have had those in excess. We shall call the red apples yang and the green apples yin.

It doesn't stop there. This time we will take away thirty green apples. What is the result? The proportion is once again lost, though this time it is not due to adding but to subtracting, generating a deficiency of green apples. We find ourselves with a relative excess of red apples, not because we've added red apples but rather because, when we took away the green apples, the red ones became the majority. They became the majority because green ones are missing, not because there is a larger quantity of red ones.

Now, so we don't start thinking this is a book about orchards and produce markets, it will be up to the reader to figure out the inverse example, when red apples are extracted and the green ones become supernumerary.

Let's go back to more typical examples:

For physiological functions (yang) to occur, nutrients (yin) are necessarily consumed. We see how yang grows at yin's expense. Likewise, the reverse: in order to absorb nutritive substances (yin), functional activity (yang) is required. Yin grows and yang diminishes (Energy is used to gain mass).

In this example we note that balance is kept in the organism when disposing of Energy and nutritive substances. But if the physiological limit of growth and decline is passed, one of the two aspects may become stronger and begin to predominate over the other, causing the latter to decline and thus making way for pathology.

As was suggested above, in reference to the ways in which yin and yang can become imbalanced, we can speak of the following syndromes:

> Cold, because yin grows
> Heat, because yang grows
> Cold, because yang diminishes
> Heat, because yin diminishes

- When a yin pathogenic factor (Cold, for example) settles in, a yin predominance is generated, damaging yang and resulting in Cold syndromes. For example, it's very cold out, we are tired, the Cold easily penetrates, and we catch a cold.
- If it is a yang pathogen, an excess of yang is produced, consuming yin, presenting Heat syndromes. A simple example is heat stroke.
- If yang diminishes, yin becomes excessive, presenting a yang deficiency. The syndrome is Cold. It is expressed as reduced yang and increased yin. To give an example that doesn't complicate things: physiological factors in the body that maintain temperature are reduced, and as a result, body temperature drops. We'll feel cold, not because the temperature around us has dropped but because of our own deficiency in the physiological regulation of our temperature.
- When there is a fluids (yin) deficiency, yang becomes excessive and appears as Heat. It is called vacant Heat because it doesn't come from an excess of yang (plenitude) but rather from a yin deficiency. For example, after profuse diarrhea, there is a reduction in body fluids.

Yin and Yang Transform into Each Other

The alternation in the growth and decline of yin and yang allows for the development of cycles. Within these cycles, when one aspect reaches its maximum expression, it begins to transform into its opposite. When the chill that starts in autumn reaches its maximum in winter, it begins to decline and little by little starts becoming Heat.

If conditions are extreme, one aspect becomes its opposite. The classic phrase reminds us of this: "Extreme yin becomes yang, and extreme yang becomes yin."

The change can occur when internal conditions and timing are ripe. We'll mention another classic example. We've already used many of these examples, but it so happens that these are the ones that appear in classical texts and illustrate the concept in clear language.

There are cases in which a person with high fever, thirst, a flushed face, and restlessness, if not treated properly, can then have a low body temperature, whose reddish complexion turns pale, and who then becomes weak and needs to be still. This is an example of how extreme yang can turn into yin.

A do-it-yourself example: prolonged contact of ice on skin will burn.

More Assessments of Yin and Yang

Yang is Movement, producing changes through action. Yin is calm and still, representing permanence. Change can be appreciated because there is something that remains still, otherwise we would have no point of reference for noticing change; we take note of the speed at which we move, among other reasons, because we perceive how we passed and left behind something that remained still.

Yang impels, creates. Yin is receptive; it is form. Yin nourishes and sustains. Yang represents a centrifugal force. Yin is a centripetal force.

Thus, yang expresses a Movement that expands from a center point out toward a periphery, in all directions. Yin corresponds with a Movement that contracts, retracts.

Yang emits; yin is the form that receives the emission. As we suggested earlier, yang is the Energy that creates, and yin is susceptible to manifesting in form or shape this impulse and creative Energy of yang.

The subtle and immaterial of yang becomes perceptible in the material of yin. The materialness of yin is organized and given a breath of Energy by yang.

In chapter 5 of *Huang Di Nei Jing,* we read: "Yin and Yang are the way of Heaven and Earth, the great outlines of everything, the parents of change, the root and beginning of birth and destruction, the palace of gods" (Lu, *A Complete Translation of The Yellow Emperor's Classic of Internal Medicine and the Difficult Classic*).

And later: "Yang is in charge of Energy transformation, and Yin is in charge of shape formation."

Heaven and Earth are representative of yin and yang. Heaven, the sky, is clear, luminous and pure, with much activity, with the Sun radiating Energy and Heat. Earth is dark, opaque, dense, receptive.

Water and Fire also teach us paradigmatic attributes of yin and yang.

Fire is warm, luminous, more immaterial, and tends to move upward.

Water is cold, damp, heavy, reflecting light but not emitting it, and slides downward.

In reference to physiological activity, functioning corresponds to yang and matter to yin.

The body's regions, Organs, and substances are assigned to yin and yang as shown in the examples in table 1.2 on page 18.

Applying Yin and Yang

Chinese Medicine is laced with notions of yin and yang. This can be observed in the classification of the organism's structures, in physiology, in pathology, and in diagnosis.

Yin yang is the guide for giving treatment and for classifying medicines and foods. But utilizing this view of opposites and its rules can be rather complicated. One must try to comprehend these notions well and practice their application as much as possible in simple day-to-day situations and from there begin to widen the scope. For deep understanding, it is necessary to persist with the intent not only to perceive from a rational standpoint but also from plain and simple sensations: feel cycles, feel opposing forces, feel transformations.

TABLE 1.2. THE BODY UNDER THE LIGHT OF YIN YANG

Yin	Yang
Lower region (below the waist)	Upper region (above the waist)
Chest and abdomen	Back
Anterior side of the limbs	Posterior side of the limbs
Organs	Viscera
Feet	Head
Internal regions (Organs)	Superficial regions (skin and muscles)
Blood	Energy
Nutritive Energy	Defensive Energy

TABLE 1.3. MANIFESTATIONS OF YIN YANG
WHEN EXAMINING PEOPLE

Examination	Yin Signs	Yang Signs
Observing	Calm, retracted, slow, seems fragile; the person is tired and weak, sleeps curled up and likes to be covered, lacks Spirit; secretions and excretions are thin and light; face is pale; tongue is swollen and damp.	Seems agitated, active, and restless; sleeps spread out, suffers insomnia, throws off blankets; fast and powerful movements; flushed; red or purple and dry tongue with thick, yellow coating.
Listening and smelling	Low, weak voice, talks little; shallow, weak, irregular breathing; sour odor.	High, rough, strong voice, talks a lot; heavy breathing; putrid odor.
Questioning	Does the person feel cold, have cold limbs and body, have little appetite, little perception of taste, prefer warm drinks, have no thirst, desire warmth and contact, have pale and abundant urine or soft stools? Does applying pressure relieve discomfort? Is menstruation scarce and light colored?	Does the person feel hot? Does heat and touch bother him or her? Are limbs and body warm? Does the person prefer cold drinks? Is the person thirsty? Constipated? Have scanty and dark urine? A dry mouth?

Data for creating table 1.3 was obtained and synthesized from *The Web That Has No Weaver,* by Ted J. Kaptchuk, and *The Foundations of Chinese Medicine,* by Giovanni Maciocia.

We saw how to apply yin yang when examining a person.

In reference to illness, yin corresponds with chronic illness, appearing gradually and evolving slowly.

Yang corresponds with acute illness, appearing suddenly and evolving quickly.

So, what about the Flowers?

Yin-Yang Flowers

Now, finally, we get to the Flowers. Here, an ocean of possibilities opens up, and clearly we will only be able to allude to a few of them, with the intent to use them in daily practice that they might propel us toward finding more applications adapted to concrete situations.

One of the first very interesting things to perceive through yin yang is the cycle of changes—the simple awareness that the tide of everything that is occurring changes. We will find both ourselves and our patients navigating with more or less ease through this sea of transformations.

When we listen to the story that the person in front of us is relaying, we may become aware of the cycles that he or she has been going through and where the person finds him- or herself in the present moment. Seeking a bit of light during dark times, discovering where we may find a bit of yang within yin in order to highlight it, we may help our patient to be nourished by it and to recover a more all-encompassing view of what is going on. And during luminous times, we may help our patient see where the seed of that which restricts Movement lies, which, at some point, will overshadow the light—the yin within yang. And then we'll work with the Flowers so that, more than words, the essences will modify these areas. We'll seek not to have a goal of holding on to just the good times but rather a goal of learning how to carve a path through the cycles.

Transformation happens in shorter or longer cycles. In knowing this, we have resources for swimming between the waves that advance and retreat. It lets us be more calm, knowing that everything comes and goes and, what is more, that we can accompany the process. And so we have at our disposal a calming factor when facing so much Movement, which is that "things will not always be like this, suffering will not persist" (unless we do everything possible to strengthen only one side of the whole). Furthermore, we have the Flowers, which open pathways and facilitate the emergence of new sentiments, thoughts, and actions, and avert stagnancy while at the same time helping us to establish our own center.

Let's take the Agrimony type or state as an example, which we will develop further in chapter 7, "The Twelve Healers." In Agrimony, it isn't too hard to notice that on the surface there is an appearance of yang—that of Movement, joy, and laughter—while internally, yin appears as worry and grief. The person is not beaming and cheerful but is also restless (often with insomnia, a tormented feeling), and this restlessness is not so obvious from the outside. The person is in Movement, unable to keep mental or physical calm. Within his or her yin, within that which is not seen from the outside, in the person's private world, there is restlessness, a facet of yang. In yin, we find yang.

There are many applications for our own lives and for therapy. Let's look at some more examples. Insisting on joy prepares a path that ends in sadness or anguish: the transformation of yang into yin. This transformation has been known since ancient times, and there are many references to cases in which it was necessary to sadden a person who was too "Vervainly" happy so that the Organs would not be affected and to prevent the person from falling into an even deeper sadness or depression. A small, inoculating sadness averts an abrupt transformation of yang to yin. We can use Vervain Flower Essence to help balance exaggerated Emotions. Scleranthus Essence can also play a part, helping the oscillations to be less marked, helping us to find our center.

Likewise, feeling sad opens a path for the arrival of joy. So it is very important to facilitate grief and to experience sorrow until the possibility is given for joy's blossoming. Holding on to sadness detains the flow of change. Protecting oneself following a maniacal bout of joy propels the cycle of transformation toward sorrow. For most of us, this is the way it goes. For those who have developed a deep understanding, there is no oscillation; when things go well, they don't get overly stirred up, and when things go poorly, they don't get markedly depressed. They know that each of these is an aspect of the whole, and it is the whole that they see. In this context, joy is not better than sorrow, nor is sorrow better than joy.

In a more general way, beginning to perceive things from yin and yang gives us a more flexible view of the world, providing more flexibility of thought and allowing us to perceive more pairs of opposites, which in itself gives us a less partial take on things, people, and processes.

Suggestions for Working with Yin Yang in Treatment

- Pay close attention to the person upon first meeting him. Our first impression can provide us with important information. Is there a tendency toward yin or yang in the way the person moves, speaks, and approaches obstacles, or in his physical appearance? Table 1.1 on page 9, showing the various expressions of yin and yang, could prove useful here.

    I remember a person who, upon arriving at my office, knocked on the door with infinite little rapid-fire knocks. Another used only two solid knocks, and another came in speaking at such a volume that, from the ground floor where we were located all the way up to the ninth floor, the neighbors noticed this person's predominant yang. Paying attention to our first impression can guide us toward one of the Twelve Healers* according to the person's yin or yang tendency. Most of all, with regard to personality type, we ought to look at the way the person exists in the world. This, of course, does not mean that we wouldn't be able to find aspects related to yang, such as anger, restlessness, anxiety, or Heat in, for example, a Mimulus type.
- Take into consideration the reason for the consultation, as it may be related to an excess or to a restriction. Being able to distinguish these aspects can orient us toward Flowers that are related with activity or passivity.
- Observe the evolution of the process. When a person with a clear yang tendency (pressured, warm, impulsive) begins showing signs of yin—but not because she is ill—she is beginning to find balance. We

---

*[Dr. Bach developed his Flower Remedies in the 1930s. He first developed the Twelve Healers, which are twelve Flowers that are related to and are used to treat twelve basic personality types, then came the Seven Helpers, followed by the last nineteen, making a total of thirty-eight Flower Remedies. —*Trans.*]

may still notice her pressured and impulsive but feeling less Heat. The pressure and impulsion will soon also probably become less marked. Likewise for someone predominantly yin who begins to show balancing signs of yang.

- Prevent the change from one extreme to the other, help bring about transformations, and avert stagnation. In some cases it is not possible to follow the flow of yin yang because there isn't enough Energy available for bringing about change. The person comprehends his situation and even has a desire to make adjustments, but there is no Energy for providing impulse. We would then say that there is stillness, a lack of Movement, in other words, a lack of yang. Flowers of great utility here are Olive, Hornbeam, and Clematis, as well as Flowers that help stop Energy drainage. Because we drain a large part of our Energy and Essence through obsessions and fixations, we can help restore Energy by recognizing obsessions and using the appropriate Flowers.

- Understand emotional and other types of changes that occur in cycles, for example, night and day.

- Observe yin-yang attributes within the Flowers themselves. Although it is possible to see pairs of opposites by comparing two related objects (like light and shadow), we can also see the yin and yang aspects of a single thing. Let's consider the Flowers: we can learn much about them when we look at them through the lens of yin yang. Let's use a Mimulus-type person as an example and, simplifying the personality, take the basic traits of fear and courage as the pair of opposites. We will seek out whatever courage the person, through her own way of existing in the world, surely possesses. Discovering and supporting this courage helps the treatment, brings forth balance, and guides our gaze toward the person's positive traits and aspects that the Flower will help to develop. This approach allows us to discover aspects of the person that were unexpected. Each Flower presents yin aspects and yang aspects, and differentiating these aspects is a worthwhile exercise. Another example of seeking the yin and yang within one Flower personality: if we perceive that the person consulting is an Impatiens type, tending toward tension and acceleration, in which ways is this person slow? It may be that his body fluids circulate at a slower-than-adequate pace. In what area of his life does he need to cooperate with others? When is he capable of being tolerant?

As we mentioned earlier, this approach is of interest because it allows us to find positive aspects and to support the development of these aspects, just as Dr. Bach suggests.

- Compare two Flowers. This is another way to learn and deepen our knowledge about the essences. Ricardo Orozco works with this approach and develops it in his book *El Nuevo Manual del Diagnóstico Diferencial de las Flores de Bach* (The New Handbook for Differential Diagnosis of Bach Flowers) about differential diagnosis.

  The comparisons stem out of yin yang. Choose two polar opposite Flowers and compare the ways in which they oppose each other and—this is very important—find how these opposites are complementary. Likewise, compare two aspects of a single Flower.

- Perceive the tendencies toward yin or yang that each Flower type presents. This can also be extended to the other groups of Flowers.

- What would happen if we saw the Virtues and defects as complementary opposites? Is it possible to uproot a defect without its corresponding Virtue also being affected?

- Be alert to what the person may be hiding. It may be helpful to be a little suspicious of our clients. If we have before us a person who is very optimistic—with an optimism that not even a Willow type can damage, nothing can take her down—our yin-yang alarm should go off. We must look for her pessimism, and we just might find a fair amount of Gentian. Obviously, the ends of our means are not to reproach her pessimism, saying, "I knew something smelled fishy," but rather to see the unseen, to see what is hidden. Yin yang guides this search.

To make sure we're on the right track, we must choose well our pair of opposites. If we are comparing two things, and for the first thing we evaluate whether it is hot or cold, and for the second we evaluate whether it is tall or short, then yes, we are comparing them, but using different pairs of opposites for each thing. We must instead use the same pair of opposites for the two things we are comparing. Let's go back to the ceiling and table example: if I view the table from the viewpoint of hot or cold, and the ceiling from the viewpoint of high or low, I'm breaking the rule of complementary opposites, and the things I'm comparing are no longer correlated.

What is more, it is most suitable to choose a pair of opposites that relate to what I'm investigating or need to find out. If I want to find out if a person is affected by cold or heat, I won't use high and low as a pair of opposites for determining whether the person is more yin or yang.

We should also perceive what is primary and what is secondary. For example, what is fundamental in the Gorse state is partial or total abandon of vitality. It is a passive attitude of retracting, retiring. Now, the person in this state may be accelerated in some aspect of his life or some physiological function, but this isn't to say that due to this yang aspect, Gorse should be cataloged as yang. Rather, we can see yang (acceleration) within yin (the Gorse state), with Yin being the primordial aspect when we study the Flower state.

Following is another important issue that obviously causes great confusion. It is quite easy to confuse the state that the Flower treats with the balancing effect that it produces. When we say Mimulus, generally we are referring to the description of the state in which a person may find herself when needing the essence. This is how it is referred to in most books on Bach Flower Remedies. We're talking about a person who is fearful, shy, restrained, with a certain level of anxiety, and not apt to share her fears and intimate concerns.

When we consult Flower Essence texts, we find a description of the state the person is in and the Flower that balances it. Regardless of the Flower we approach, these are the types of descriptions we read. In other words, we are told what imbalance the Flower Essence treats.

If we read the section that talks about the positive aspects related to the Flower, we are then touching on the effect that the essence can provoke.

Continuing with Mimulus, the essence helps one feel more confident, less timid, be more active, have more courage, and feel more free. When viewed from the viewpoint of yin yang, the Mimulus state that the person expresses has a Yin tendency, while the effect that the essence provides leads toward yang. We can then say that Mimulus Flower Essence, when taken, leads to yang, thus balancing the yin tendency that people in Mimulus states tend to exhibit.

Much disorientation and lengthy discussions will ensue if we don't take into account these differences. Knowing what it is I'm referring to, whether I am talking about the state of the person herself (fear, sadness, and so on, according to the essence in question) or speaking of the balancing effect that the essence brings about, are very important differences when applying yin yang.

For continued study of yin yang, consult the bibliography of this book and allow what you read to settle in and blossom forth in perceptions and day-to-day applications.

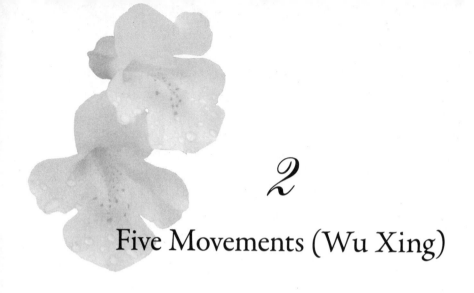

2

Five Movements (Wu Xing)

*T*he sages of ancient times denominated as yin and yang the two aspects that Energy takes on in the process of becoming manifest. In the previous chapter, we mentioned that forms and multiplicity emerge out of the interaction between yin and yang.

In the cycles of yin's and yang's growth and decline, Energy takes on specific characteristics. There are five of these dynamic phases. Thanks to the movements and changes of these phases, each thing in the world enters into existence. These five phases also mark the natural transformations that every being and process in the manifest world is exposed to.

Each one of these Movements has distinguishing qualities and each receives a name. They are called Water, Wood, Fire, Earth, and Metal. We will approach these characteristics by looking at the following cycle of movement:

- We are still.
- We begin walking, and the movement gradually becomes faster.
- We reach what we consider our top speed at the time.
- We maintain the speed of this movement.
- We begin reducing the speed of our movement, and it gradually slows.
- Movement ceases, and we return to stillness.

With this, we have an inkling about the quality of each phase, expressed in terms of movement.

We will begin our tour with the distinctive features of the Water Movement, followed by Wood, Fire, Earth, Metal, and, finally, the return to Water. In Water we find ourselves in a period of rest and reserve; in Wood, Energy begins to unfurl, reaching its maximum expression in Fire, sustained by Earth; and then in Metal, it begins deceleration as the impulse of Energy decreases until once again it finds stillness where it is amassed.

Having recognized the dynamic nature of the Five Movements, let's devote some time to getting to know other aspects.

- The Five Movements allow us to classify objects and phenomena into five categories.
- They express the five ways in which nature manifests itself.
- They also show us, through the bonds they maintain among one another, relationships and dynamics of objects and phenomena in our manifest world.
- They were originally about five substances, and like yin and yang, the meaning of these natural substances grew to symbolize Energy's cycles of change.

Characteristics of the Five Movements

In texts from various eras explaining this part of Chinese Medicine, it is common to find the following way of describing the characteristics of each Movement. Although some of the phrases may seem repetitive, I have included them because their symbolic and evocative richness may awaken in the reader associations both with the Flowers and with other aspects of Flower Essence Therapy.

Wood
It grows upward and expands outward.
Growth, externalization, and expansion.
Flexibility, vital impulse, free Movement.
It can be bent and straightened.
Flexible and tenacious upward growth.
It may seem as if its life were weak, but no force can destroy it.
It is soft and seeks to grow freely.

Fire

It flames and moves upward.

Warming and ascending.

Production of Heat and ascending Movement.

It guarantees robust growth of all things in nature. The Heart's Energy
is alive and restless.

Earth

Going to seed; gathering.

Production, support, reception.

Transformation, transport of fluids and nutritive elements.

Sowing, growth, and harvest.

It is solid and still, able to hold and to nourish all things.

Fertility.

Metal

Operator of change and reform.

Purification, internalization, retraction.

Malleability and hardness: it can be modeled and hardened.

Rigor: it can cut, prune, and reduce.

Gather, collect, whittle down to that which is essential.

Clear and cool, it can make an impression of severity, like the autumn
wind that dries up the grass and leaves.

Purity and firmness.

Water

It moistens and is filtered downward.

Cooling, moistening, descent.

Accumulation that stagnates.

Conservation, amassing.

It is calm and cold.

Lubrication.

Any thing, situation, phenomenon, or person with characteristics
that can be associated with a Movement is assigned to it. Let's look at
this example: anything that tends to move downward, is cold, and stagnates can be associated with Water. Winter, which is the season corre-

sponding with Water, exhibits these characteristics. At this time of year, Energy tends to move toward the center of the Earth, and everything slows down, stagnates, freezes.

Correlations

We've stated that through the theory of the Five Movements we can classify things. In table 2.1 (on page 31), we'll see some of the classifications related with the Five Movements, both in nature and in relation to the human being. Based on Energy's characteristics in each Movement, we can also appreciate the unity between human beings and the cosmos; in a single current, a Movement unites aspects of the human being with aspects of nature. For example, when we say Liver, anger, Jupiter, Wind, spring, and dawn, we are speaking of Wood. All the aspects mentioned cease to be unrelated and are united under the qualities of Wood. Seeing things under this light opens the door to comprehending an amazing number of relationships.

The time has come to clarify that the relationships and classifications that the Five Movements emphasize are not absolute, in the sense that they do not completely and totally explain in every situation the functioning of the universe and of human beings. Nevertheless, they are applicable and allow us access to very valuable information. If we use the Five Movements theory—and the information we obtain by applying it—with flexibility and in conjunction with other elements at our disposal as Flower Essence Therapists and practitioners of Chinese Medicine, our work will be notably enriched.

We'll broaden the subject when we get into the Emotions and their relationships with the internal Organs in chapter 5.

For those of us who practice Flower Essence Therapy, applying these correlations may be a great opportunity for asking questions during consultations, questions that can serve as triggers and lead to various issues, creating openness.

Something else we must take into consideration is that openness, and thus the possibility for deepening our work with our clients, will be very difficult if we use our knowledge of the correlations in the Five Movements for dictating sentences, taking everything for granted, and sticking everything—people and their attitudes—into little boxes. In short, believing we know who and how the other person is. We must, with the other person during consultations, put into play the relationships that we are able to establish and the information we are able to obtain in order to adjust these to the peculiarities of each person. Here lies the art of their application.

It's advisable to avoid the strict application of this knowledge or to use it as a means for wielding power. We would do very well to not give in to the temptation of believing that everything is a perfectly assembled machine, of believing that since this is the way it is, I can work it like a production line, as in "Ah, here comes a lady from the A5 series—great, I know the drill so here are the Flowers." Although this approach may seem comfortable and reassuring for the therapist, it is not at all advisable, either for the patient or for the work the two will carry out together.

Further ahead, when referring to suggestions for applying the Five Movements theory, we'll talk about some ways to use these correspondences in relation to the Flowers.

Relationships between the Five Movements

The Five Movements are not isolated compartments; instead, they maintain relationships with one another. Because they represent phases of change in Energy, they are interdependent; each one of these Movements is dynamically intertwined with the others, one following the other in a harmonic order (in Chinese Medicine texts this is called a physiological order) and a discordant order (called a pathological order).

We find two cycles that express harmonious relationships between the Five Movements: the Generating Cycle and the Dominating Cycle.

The Generating Cycle
Each Movement engenders another, nourishing it and favoring its growth, and at the same time, each Movement is engendered by another. This cycle has been called the mother-son cycle, therefore:

Wood is the mother of Fire.
Fire engenders Earth.
Earth gives rise to Metal.

TABLE 2.1. CORRESPONDENCES AMONG
THE FIVE MOVEMENTS

Five Movements	Wood	Fire	Earth	Metal	Water
Planet	Jupiter	Mars	Saturn	Venus	Mercury
Direction	East	South	Center	West	North
Color	Blue-green	Red	Yellow	White	Black
Climate	Wind	Heat	Damp	Dry	Cold
Season	Spring	Summer	End of summer	Autumn	Winter
Time of Day	Dawn	Midday	Afternoon	Sunset	Midnight
Developmental Stages	Birth Engendering	Growth	Plenitude Transformation	Decline Seed-saving Harvest	Death Conservation Storage
Organs	Liver	Heart	Spleen	Lung	Kidney
Viscera	Gallbladder	Small Intestine	Stomach	Large Intestine	Bladder
Sensory Organs	Eyes	Tongue	Mouth	Nose	Ears
Senses	Sight	Word	Touch	Smell	Hearing
Fluids	Tears	Sweat	Thin saliva (drool)	Mucus	Thick saliva
Flavors	Sour	Bitter	Sweet	Pungent	Salty
Tissues	Tendons	Arteries Blood vessels	Muscles Flesh Limbs	Skin	Bones Teeth
Appears In	Fingernails	Pulse Complexion	Lips	Body hair	Hair (on head)
Expressions	Shouting	Laughter	Song	Crying	Moaning Groaning
Emotions	Anger Irritability	Joy Scare/ surprise	Worry Meditation Anxiety Nostalgia Reflection	Anguish Sadness Unsettled	Fear Insanity
Psyches	Hun	Shen	Yi	Po	Zhi
Scents	Rancid	Burnt	Fragrant Aromatic Perfumed	Animal decomposition	Rotten Fermented
Ways of Reacting	Clenching fists	Dejection Upset	Belching Vomiting	Coughing Expectorating	Trembling Shivers
Virtues	Kindness Benevolence	Courtesy Correctness	Confidence Faith	Justice Rectitude	Intelligence Wisdom
Effort	Ocular abuse	Excessive walking	Abuse of the seated position	Abuse of the reclined position	Abuse of the standing position

> Metal gives life to Water.
> Water generates Wood.

Thus, the activation and growth of each Movement is produced. Energy circulates in an uninterrupted cycle, passing from mother to son.

If this were the only relationship, growth would become exaggerated and harmful. Indefinite expansion ultimately leads to dispersion.

The Dominating Cycle averts the limitless growth of each Movement, providing opposition that brings balance.

The Dominating Cycle

Each Movement controls, restrains, and contains the development of another and at the same time is, itself, controlled by another. So, in this way:

> Wood controls Earth.
> Earth controls Water.
> Water controls Fire.
> Fire controls Metal.
> Metal controls Wood.

We can see, then, that each Movement is generated by and generates another and is dominated by and dominates another. To give an example: Fire is the son of Wood and the mother of Earth; it dominates Metal and is dominated by Water.

A dominating Movement in the Dominating Cycle not only averts an overflowing of the Movement it dominates but also helps it to carry out its function.

These relationships help us understand transformations occurring in nature and in human beings: relationships between internal Organs, Emotions, physiological processes, and so on.

The Generating and Dominating Cycles show us balanced and harmonious proportions in the relationships between the Five Movements. The Oppression and Opposition Cycles represent distorted relationships where proportion is lost.

The Oppression Cycle

This cycle is an abuse of what happens in the Dominating Cycle. At some point, the dominating Movement may be in excess, or the dominated Movement may be weak. These circumstances set the stage for what we might call an abuse of power by the dominating Movement.

The Oppression Cycle follows the same circuit as the Dominating Cycle.

The help and support given in the Dominating Cycle are lost and instead of favoring the dominated Movement's tasks, it oppresses and restricts, stunting that Movement's work.

So for example, Metal might excessively dominate Wood or take advantage of a weakness in Wood.

The Opposition Cycle

This cycle expresses how a Movement turns against the one dominating it, inverting the Dominating Cycle into one of counterdomination or opposition.

So Water rebels against Earth, which is the Movement that, in the context of a balanced expression of the cycles, would dominate it. In this situation, the imbalance is serious and tends to get worse.

It is recommended to learn and retain the relationships between the Five Movements, as they help us to comprehend many aspects of Chinese Medicine, including what is written in textbooks and in classical texts. For example, when studying the effect the excess consumption of a flavor has on the body's tissues, we are looking at a Dominating Cycle. So, excess sweets (the flavor corresponding with the Earth Movement) generates disorders in areas related to Water, as Water is the Movement that dominates Earth. We would then see issues in the person's bones, teeth, and possibly hair. So we see that, thanks to the Dominating Cycle, we can foresee what areas will be affected when one eats too many sweet-flavored foods. What is more, bringing our attention to the relationship between bones and sweet-flavored foods, we realize that in a disorder as common these days as osteoporosis, not only is it important to increase calcium (and other minerals), but we may also need to regulate the consumption of sweet-flavored foods, something that is not usually taken into consideration in therapeutic practice. In these moments of realization, we may suddenly appreciate the work of so many wise people over the centuries.

Viewing the Movements' Interrelatedness from the Position of Metal

What we've mentioned is just one example of the infinite possibilities for applying the Five Movements theory. To continue understanding these relationships, let's focus on one Movement, as we've done in previous pages. In this case, let's look at Metal.

> Metal is the son of Earth.
> It is the mother of Water.
> It dominates Wood.
> It is dominated by Fire.

Using this example, we see that each Movement maintains relationships with the other four, carrying out different roles. The mother of a Movement in one case dominates a Movement in another case and so on. Therefore we acknowledge that a fixed role cannot be assigned to each Movement and that its function depends upon the relationship it maintains with whichever other Movement it is joined with at the time. Here's an example using colors: if we take green and put it next to red, the two give off a sensation that you don't have to be an expert in fine art to notice. This same green color put next to purple impacts us in a different way, and when put next to black, everything changes once again. It is the same green color, but its function, what it transmits and how it vibrates, changes according to the relationship it establishes with other colors. What determines the role is the relationship, meaning, and place that a particular Movement occupies at any given time. In other words, the role is not determined by the individual Movement but rather by the relationship it establishes.

Each Movement carries out all the functions, and thus the Movements balance each other, keeping circulation and transformation of Energy in harmony.

What happens when a Movement is too powerful? It is going to oppress the one it dominates and turn against the one that dominates it.

If Metal is excessively forceful,

> it oppresses Wood
> it turns against Fire

And if Metal is weak,

> Fire oppresses it
> Wood turns against it

How Energy Is Expressed in Each Movement

All this turns out to be pretty interesting once we comprehend how Energy moves when it manifests itself in a determined Movement and the relationships that arise among them due to the characteristics of Energy's Movement style in each.

Wood: Energy has serious strength, expanding in all directions. It seeks externalization. It grows upward.
Fire: Energy moves vigorously upward.
Earth: Energy spins horizontally around its own axis.
Metal: Energy moves inward. It retracts, condenses, and tends to become compact.
Water: Energy moves downward.

Now that we have an idea of each Movement's characteristics, and keeping in mind the sort of impulse of each and in which direction Energy moves in each, let's now look at the relationships among them. To look at the cycle of Energy transformation, we'll begin with Water.

- When Energy is in **Water**, it tends to be still, storing itself up like a treasure and regenerating itself so that another cycle of transformation may begin. It is the moment of quietude, before initiating Movement, a preparation for the impulse to start. Thus it gives birth to Wood's creative force. The descending momentum of Energy during its Water phase incites Wood's expansive upward and outward Movement.
- Movement is now initiated in **Wood**, with the strength of something wanting to be born, to burst into the world. Development begins. Movement is expansive, explosive. That which was in repose, hidden, now shows itself outwardly. The impulse that Energy has in Wood initiates a Movement that will take on its full expression in Fire.
- **Fire** reveals the expansive and externalized Movement of that which has reached its plenitude and maximum expression. Energy is agitated

and projects itself powerfully upward. We noted in the chapter about yin yang, in reference to intertransformation, that yin becomes yang and yang becomes yin. During the Fire phase, we are present to the transformation of yang into yin, mediated by Earth's Movement, which will prevent the change from being too abrupt. Having reached its maximum expression and Movement, Energy in the Fire phase begins to seek quietude, diminishing its impulse. Fire's own impetus incites Earth's strength, capable of modulating the upward fugue of Fire Energy. Energy cannot continue its growth; it begins its return.

- Having reached the **Earth** phase, the ascending and expansive impulse turns into a Movement that spins around itself, neither continuing to grow nor stopping or descending. It is a transitional phase, of balance before change, before yin begins to grow. Earth receives Fire's Energy, transforms it, and adjusts it, converting it into Metal Energy. When Earth Energy is potent, so too will be Metal's contracting impulse.

- **Metal** receives Earth's revolving Energy, thus beginning the phase of contraction, as Energy moves toward center. It is the time for return; the transformative journey that Energy has been making is coming to a close. A return to the starting point is being imposed. Energy becomes denser. By transforming the revolving Energy expressed in Earth into a Movement of condensation, the path is cleared so that Energy can take on the descending direction of Water, whose strength depends on the centripetal force of Metal's Movement of Energy.

- Back to **Water**. The full cycle of Energy's transformation has been fulfilled through the phases of yin's and yang's growth and decline. If Water's capacity to amass and regenerate Energy—to keep life in waiting, like it does in winter—lacks strength, its transmission to Wood will be weak. Consequently, Wood will have less potency. The same thing will happen if the descending force of Water is weak. What is more, as Water represents the end of the cycle and a new beginning, the entire next cycle will be affected.

Following the transformation of Energy, in the cycle we just observed, we can see that

- from Water to Fire, yang grows, and from Fire to Water, yin grows
- from Water to Fire, yin decreases, and from Fire to Water, yang decreases

Keeping Balance: Mutual Support
among the Movements

Water. The descending force that Energy expresses during this phase balances the ascending Energy of Fire. If Water's action is weak, Fire lacks a counterweight, so there is nothing to stop its Energy from shooting upward and becoming dispersed, debasing its task and breaking the balance. Water represents coolness, preventing excess Heat from Fire. So in the body, the equivalent of a weakness in Water's action could be Heat drying up body fluids.

If Water is too powerful, it could excessively chill and extinguish Fire.

Wood. The incitement of Wood's expansive Movement helps prevent Earth Energy from exaggerating its characteristic Movement of spinning on its axis. Wood prevents Earth from closing in on itself, in which case it would run the risk of slowing impulse enough to stop impulse entirely.

Weakness in Wood's force allows Earth Energy to stifle and deteriorate Wood's dynamism.

If Wood Energy is too pushy, it subverts and disturbs Earth, negatively influencing Earth's operative capacity.

Fire. It supports Metal Energy, helping it to not become too solid and cold. It modulates Metal Energy's contracting force.

Debilitated Fire Energy favors the rigidity of Metal, diminishing its capacity for adaptation.

If Fire's potency is exaggerated, Metal loses its shape, becoming too malleable.

Earth. Thanks to its revolving Energy, Earth regulates the descending impulse of Water's Energy.

When Earth is weak, Water increases its capacity to sink into the depths.

The excessive action of Earth Energy makes descent difficult, favoring accumulation.

Metal. The collaboration that Metal offers Wood is that of modulating its characteristic expansive, ascending Energy. The contracting Movement of Metal balances the expansive Energy of Wood.

If Metal is weak, Wood becomes too powerful and can destroy everything.

If Metal's force is too powerful, it can excessively restrict the Movement, expansion, and growth of Wood.

Earth is key.

This Movement, because of its characteristics, is the great harmonizer of all the elements. This will be easier to see when we assess Earth's position in figure 2.1.

Earth, in the center, equidistant from the other Movements, creates a nucleus for the others, bringing unity to the whole system. Earth prevents the other Movements from becoming scattered. It balances Fire's ascending Movement and Water's descending Movement, as it does Wood's expansive Movement and Metal's contracting Movement.

Energy's way of behaving, along with each Movement's characteristics, creates an ocean of possibilities in relation to the Flowers. A minimal example: Wood's expansiveness and Fire's plenitude, both of which can easily be exaggerated, bring to mind Vervain, whose manner of being in the world can be understood in the context of these two Movements. Once this relationship is verified, we'll investigate Fire- and Wood-related aspects in a markedly Vervain-type person: the Organs, tissues, and Emotions that are implicated, among other aspects.

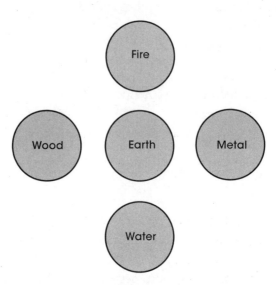

Figure 2.1. Earth as the harmonizer among the Five Movements

Beginning to Establish
Relationships

We stated that everything sharing the characteristics of a determined Movement can be classified under the ranks of that Movement. The paragraphs we developed regarding Energy's Movements, according to the Five Movements and their relationships and characteristics, allow us to comprehend many of the assignments of an Organ, tissue, person, thing, occurrence, and so on to a particular Movement.

In Chinese Medicine, each one of the Five Organs (Liver, Heart, Spleen, Lung, and Kidney) corresponds with a Movement, because its physiological function is analogous to the characteristics of the Movement to which it is assigned. (Consult correspondences in table 2.1 on page 31.)

The correspondences between a Movement and an Organ also extend to the related tissues, sensory Organs, Viscera, body fluids, and so on (see figure 2.2). Likewise, these relationships cover the Emotions and the Psyches, which, by being related to the Organs, not only demonstrate the integrity of the human being's processes and substrata but also lay out a world of relationships between the Organs, Emotions, Psyches, and, through the Organs, their entire area of influence in the body. They are paths that cross, allowing passage from the Emotions to the body, to the Psyche, to the Organs.

Thus we can comprehend how a Flower Essence's action can influence a determined Organ or tissue. By using the Flowers, it is also

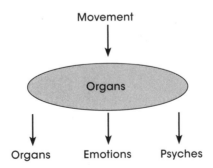

*Figure 2.2. Correspondences between a Movement and its
Organ and related Emotions, Organs, and Psyches*

possible for us to adjust emotional dynamics, the Psyches, the influence of these on the Organs, and, as such, the related territories in the body.

Through the Transpersonal Patterns developed by Ricardo Orozco, our prospects open even wider for linking the Flowers with the world of relationships we've just outlined.

Applications in the Area of Chinese Medicine

- The Five Movements allow us to observe the integration of the organism's various structures and functions.
- The physiological functioning of the Organs and Viscera can be explained according to the characteristics of each Movement.
- The physiological relationships between Organs and Viscera can be viewed under the light of the Generating Cycle and Dominating Cycle.
- Pathological relationships may also be studied from this perspective, observing, for example, how imbalances evolve and move through the system following the different cycles.
- The Five Movements give us prospects for diagnosis as well as orienting principles for treatment.

There is a wide range of applications for this medicine. Take into consideration that the yin yang and *Wu Xing* (Five Movements) theories are the pillars of Chinese Medicine.

Some of these applications may be of great use for our work with the Flowers. One of these may be the transmission and evolution of imbalances.

The Five Movements theory gives us a model for understanding how imbalances might evolve and change. The relationships between the Five Movements show us paths through which disorders may develop. The transmission of disorders may take different routes according to the different cycles.

In order to better follow what is about to be explained, it would be helpful to have handy the diagram of the Five Movements and their relationships (figure 2.3).

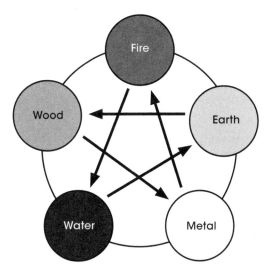

Figure 2.3. The Five Movements and their relationships

By Way of the Generating Cycle
- The mother's imbalance is passed to the son.
  The mother Movement does not nourish the son.
  If Water is deficient, it cannot nourish Wood.
- The son's imbalance is passed to the mother.
  The son Movement exhausts its mother.
  Fire exhausts Wood.

By Way of the Oppression Cycle
- The Movement that dominates is too forceful.
  Wood oppresses Earth.
- The oppressed Movement is weak.
  Earth is weak, inciting Wood to oppress it.

By Way of the Opposition Cycle
- The dominating Movement is weak.
  Metal lacks strength; Wood suppresses it.
- The Movement that is dominated lacks strength.
  Fire is too forceful and turns against Water.

When a Movement Is Weak

We must look for where there is excess.

The weakened Movement could be getting oppressed by the one dominating it, and there we find the excess. It could also be that the weakened Movement is being opposed by the Movement that it should be dominating.

Fire is weak. Water probably has too much Energy, and Metal is "taking advantage of" Fire's weakness, oppressing it.

When a Movement Is Excessively Forceful

A Movement exhibiting excess Energy tends to oppress the one it dominates and oppose the Movement that dominates it. Metal is too forceful, opposing Wood and oppressing Fire.

Another View

One of my teachers and friends, Ricardo Fernández Herrero, maintains that when a Movement is in excess it interrupts the transmission of Energy to its son and reroutes it toward the Movement that dominates it, thereby opposing it.

Earth in excess stops supplying Energy to Metal and opposes Water.

So the whole dynamic of the Movements becomes unbalanced. Imagine what happens when the son of a Movement that is in excess stops being nourished. It loses strength, and because it is unable to nourish its own son, the domination function fails.

The Five Movements can orient us when evaluating our client's motive for consulting us. They help steer our work with the person and help us to create strategies for treatment.

Suggestions for Working with Clients

Emotions

Although we will talk about Emotions in chapter 3, the correlations that can be established based on the relationships between the Organs, their spheres of influence, and the Emotions are enormously useful, so we will go ahead and mention them. It is equally important to understand that Emotions affect the whole body, the entirety of the person, and that the correlation between an Emotion and an Organ is not something rigid but rather a reference point, allowing us to investigate. When we give our client a Flower that balances an Emotion, we are favoring balance in the related Organ.

For example, anger injures the Liver, generating dysfunction. By using Holly Flower Essence, we are bringing harmony to this Organ; through the regulation of anger, we are indirectly improving the Liver's functioning.

What is more, any Liver disorder can find relief when anger is not also pressuring it and provoking its malfunction. So using Flower Essences can help prevent anger, as a pathogenic factor, from affecting the Liver. On the other hand, this Emotion could worsen any disorders that the Liver and its areas of influence might be suffering.

An Organ and Its Area of Influence

Now we'll go from disorders in some part of the body to the Emotions. Because of the correspondences of the Five Movements, we know that muscles are an area influenced by Earth via the Spleen. If muscle tone is upset, or if there is weakness in the limbs, we might ask about nostalgia and excessive mental activity, such as a lot of studying or a lot of thinking about some topic. Likewise, we will look at what's going on with an obsessive type of person with a fixation on some issue.

The Psyches

There will also be a chapter about the Psyches. For now we will say that, as with the Emotions, the Psyches associated with a Movement, and thus with an Organ, can indicate dysfunctions in an Organ and its areas of influence. Likewise, the reverse: a disturbance in a tissue or body part will lead us to consider aspects of the related Organ's Psyche.

Prevention

Knowing the relationships between the Emotions, Organs, Psyches, and different regions of the body allows us to see how deep the imbalance has become. We can see which group of Emotions is implicated, and whether the imbalance remains at the Emotional and Psyche levels or if it has evolved into the body.

Earlier, we talked about the transmission of disorders, and we can use this aspect of the Five Movements for prevention. Let's look at a basic example: when we perceive that the imbalance is in a certain Movement, we will take special care of the Movement that is dominated by the affected one. If Fire is upset, we will pay special attention to Metal in order to strengthen it and prevent the disorder from being transmitted to it.

For our work with the Flowers, we can view this approach by focusing on the Emotions. Using the example given above, we will try to keep Metal (the Lung) from being weakened by sadness. This is how we could strengthen it. Knowing that anguish as well as sadness affect the Lung, which corresponds to Metal, we have Mustard and Sweet Chestnut at hand. Staying alert and not letting Metal become affected by way of disturbances in its Psyche, we favor adaptation to change. Imagine a markedly Rock Water–type person who finds himself in the above situation. On the one hand, a little Heat from Fire would do him some good to loosen up some of the rigidity, but an excess or deficiency in Fire would disturb him, and he would feel more insecure, or more rigid and less flexible. This is why, knowing that there are disorders in Fire, we will try to favor Metal's harmonious functioning. This may prove to be relatively simple or more complicated depending on the circumstances and on the person's Flower-type tendencies. Treating a Rock Water type is not the same as treating an Impatiens, Vervain, or Mimulus type. Each one of these Flower types will make us attentive to different aspects of Metal. In Mimulus, for example, we would try to prevent further retraction because we know that it would create an imbalance in Metal whose energetic Movement is already one of contracting and of slowing impulse. On the other hand, a Vervain type would create imbalances in Metal by pushing every limit.

Evolution of Treatment

Data recorded in ancient texts already tell us that if imbalances are transmitted through the Generating Cycle, from mother to son, they turn out to be less severe than if they are transmitted from son to mother.

The same thing happens via the Dominating Cycle: disorders are less severe by domination than by opposition (when the dominated Movement opposes he who dominates it). Without taking this as absolute truth, and much less as a death sentence, we might orient ourselves by viewing this from the perspective of the Emotions. Let's take fear (corresponding to Water). If a person who has been feeling fear for a long time begins to feel sadness (corresponding to Metal) and that Emotion sets in, we'll want to watch out for evolution in the situation that is not particularly positive. If, on the other hand, fear passes into anger (corresponding to Wood), the Movement of the Emotions follows the Generating Cycle, and as follows, we would be observing a positive evolution. We're not talking about Emotions that arise, are felt, and then move on, as these are not chronic or long-standing.

So we notice that a Movement is affected by disorders in its incumbent Emotions, or by imbalances in its associated Organs, body regions, and Psyches. These are indicators that guide us and lead us to inquire, to work with the person who is consulting us, as it is within this shared work that the data obtained takes on meaning and truth.

Relationships between the Five Movements

When an Emotion settles in and stays awhile, we might view it under the light of the relationships between the Five Movements.

Resentment indicates a Wood-related disorder, so we will take this Movement as a point of reference. We'll check to see if there are other ailments at other levels (like in the body) of this same Movement. We will also try to perceive what is happening in the areas of: Metal (sadness), which dominates Wood; Earth (nostalgia, worry), which is dominated by Wood; Fire (joy, excitement), which is the son; and Water (fear, fright), which is the mother.

This way we will be able to detect if another Movement is influencing Wood in such a way that regulating resentment becomes more difficult. Likewise, to detect if the imbalance in Wood is obstructing other Movements' performance. So by regulating the Emotions associated with other Movements that are found to be out of balance, we are favoring a harmony that will help to resolve resentment. Obviously, the person will have to do her part, but the path will be cleared for her to do it. For example, by adjusting Earth-related Emotions (nostalgia, excess reflection, worry), we improve the prospects for resolving resentment. The stagnation and mucus that may be generated by a poorly functioning Spleen (corresponding to Earth) provide a base for resentment to become chronic. Earth endangers Wood (Oppression Cycle). At the same time, people who hold resentment for a long time will have tendencies toward stagnation, generating mucus, and a lagging circulation of body fluids (Wood out of balance affects Earth). I have observed sluggish lymphatic circulation and mucus accumulation in people with old resentments.

It can be useful to ask which disorders appeared first in order to observe the evolution of the imbalance. In Chinese Medicine, there are principles for treatment based on the relationships between the Five Movements.

Another way to work with these relationships is to detect imbalances and then support the development of the Movement that will bring balance, by cultivating harmony in the associated Emotions as well as a balanced expression of the Psyche, which provides Virtues.

Let's say that Metal is the Movement that's out of balance, expressed in the form of serious sadness. We will seek to develop Fire's Movement to bring about joy by using whichever essences we believe to be most appropriate. Letting ourselves be guided by the defects and Virtues of the Twelve Healers, we might propose Water Violet, whose Virtue is joy. This way we are not focusing only on sadness. We would seek to balance Fire-related aspects to help Fire fulfill its function of modulating Metal, for example by avoiding frivolous excitement, acceleration, and stimulus. To nourish Metal, we would support a balanced Earth Movement by adjusting nostalgia and worry for example. We would accomplish this by giving essences and also by recommending tasks and attitudes associated with the Movement that regulate the imbalance. As we get further along in the book, we will gain more clarity for how to go about doing this.

Relationships with Nature

Colors, times of day, flavors, and climate associated with a Movement are elements containing important data. For example, a green tinge to the skin (green corresponds to Wood) may indicate Liver disorders. We would think of anger. Flavors also indicate a possible imbalance in a Movement. Sour corresponds to Wood, so if a person particularly likes or dislikes that flavor, we would investigate imbalances in Wood's sphere of influence.

One of these pieces of information on its own does not qualify us to be categorical in an evaluation. We must combine the information we receive with other information from our evaluation, whether it comes from knowledge related to Bach Flower Therapy or knowledge that comes from resources based in Chinese Medicine.

How to Help Treatment Along

When we know which Emotion, Psyche, or body region and tissue may be affected, we can take steps to help recover balance. Continuing with Wood, when this Movement is affected, overuse of eyesight is not recommended, especially at night. In the case of a pregnant woman, it is particularly advisable to pay close attention to these suggestions.

It will also be useful to know which flavors harm the treatment's evolution. In Wood's case, the absence or excess of sour flavors does not help, and excess pungent flavors will create further imbalance. So we see that pungent flavors could interfere negatively when we are trying to modulate anger.

The Cycle

The Generating Cycle can be applied in a variety of circumstances.

One way to apply it is to look at one whole cycle as life's Movement through different phases.

We begin in Water, an undifferentiated state. We are born in Wood, and our development and growth unfolds during Fire. We reach adulthood during Earth, old age during Metal, and in death, we return, once again, to Water.

A person may go through this entire cycle and never learn a thing. Or try to avoid the whole thing and return quickly, as is Clematis's case, eager to return to the beginning without ever fully immersing herself in life to carry out the whole cycle with its inherent opportunities for learning.

A person could remain stuck in a certain Movement despite the passage of time. For example, Fire, forever young, denies the passage of time, hoping to ride the crest of the energetic wave forever. So, what was it like during each phase for the person consulting us? Was he able to push forth with Wood's Energy? Even though it is an expansive phase, did he have to restrain himself? How are those circumstances playing out now that he is passing through the Earth phase? What are the effects? Francesc Mariegas's work with the Five Movements in relation to self-awareness and evolution is excellent, both in its astounding theory and its practice. His book, *El Tao del Cambio* (The Dao of Change), is a huge contribution to our work with Flower Essence Therapy.

The same cycle can be applied to understand how the person behaves in different phases of an undertaking. Is it hard for her to begin (Wood), or do things get complicated at the end (Water)? What happens when it comes time for her to sustain what she's attained? And when it's time to harvest the fruits of her labor?

We repeatedly find clients with problems during one of these phases, and many times the person hasn't even noticed it. We can clear stagnation with Flower Essences and with other aspects related to an imbalanced Movement and its relationship with the other Movements. If a person has a hard time starting things, we'll take a look at how he manages the endings of things. We'll see if trouble starting things is due to acceleration and excessive expansion, or if it is a lack of impulse due to retraction and restriction (Wood may be weak, and/or Metal may be very forceful).

Characteristics of the Movements and Individuals

Individuals tend to express their vitality through one of the Five Movements. If we have before us someone who tends to express herself through Wood, she will do so impulsively, in a way that is expansive, and when imbalanced she will become invasive. This will give us guidelines about how she accumulates and drains Energy, which errors she tends to make, and what causes her suffering, all of which can be worked on with the Flowers.

This viewpoint is expanded and enriched when we add in the Psyches, Emotions, and Organs.

Learning and the Way One Tends to Exist in the World

This point is closely related with the previous point about a person's characteristics. As Eduardo Alexander tells us in his thesis "Nutrindo a vitalidade" (Nourishing Vitality), at some point early on in life, something happened (probably traumatic) that left us processing the world from one fixed viewpoint. We view the world from one of the Movements. We tend then to interpret everything that happens to us and in general from that viewpoint. This circumstance leads to an accumulation of Energy in the Movement of our fixation, generating weakness in the others. The Emotions, Psyches, and physical disorders are a guide to help us discover which Movement we prioritize when we process whatever comes our way. When we identify it, we can begin to develop the Virtues associated with that Movement as a way of deconstructing our interpretive rigidity. The Flowers are one of the most appropriate tools for cultivating Virtues. We will soon see why.

These are just a few of the applications that the Five Movements offer us. Possibly the easiest way to begin is to use the correspondences for establishing relationships between Organs, Emotions, Psyches, and body regions and tissues.

The Emotions and Psyches provide us with tools that are not far from our work as Bach Flower Therapists. Perceiving the Emotions in the person consulting us, observing which Psyches are imbalanced, and giving the corresponding Flower Essences could be within the abilities of every Flower Essence Therapist. It is a way to organize the information that we know how to obtain through our training as therapists.

The Five Movements allow us to see the storyline that unifies the various bits of information we acquire and to integrate them, deepening and widening our comprehension, bringing us to treatment possibilities that we otherwise might not have imagined.

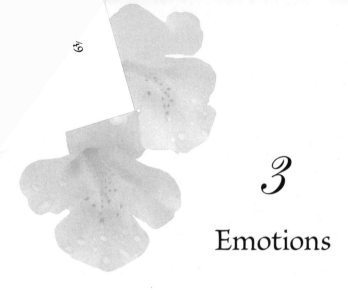

3

Emotions

*W*e are immersed in emotions as if swimming in an ocean. When we as Flower Essence Therapists are visiting with clients, emotions are often the nexus that bring us to the Flower Remedies. Along with thoughts, emotions can be the guiding compass that shows us how the person exists in the world and, as such, how he reacts to life's incidents, including illness. Emotions can also give us clues as to the defects and Virtues needing work, as we'll see in chapter 6.

The space that Chinese Medicine gives to emotions may be of great interest to us in our work with the Flowers.

If we go a little further back in time, before Chinese Medicine arose, and view emotions from the Daoist perspective, these arise when Energy leaves *center* and ascends to the head. On its journey upward, Energy manifests itself as emotion.

When yin and yang separate and we no longer exist in unity, the Five Movements lose their natural shape and are no longer expressed through the Five Virtues but rather as the Five Emotions—and so the dance begins.

Within Chinese Medicine's conceptual framework of the causes of illness, Emotions are considered internal causes. They are also called internal injuries and can directly affect the Organs. To consider Emotions as something generating internal injuries is quite a stance to take.

Emotions in order to "injure" and thus constitute a cause of illness must fulfill certain criteria:

> They must be very strong.
> They must be raw.
> They must persist over time.
> They must be repeated.

If they fall into these parameters, they'll manage to upset Blood and Energy and the circulatory mechanisms of both.

We can already begin to apply this knowledge in our practice by registering the Emotions that get repeated, not only during the consultation but also those that insist on coming up periodically, as well as those that persist, as these may be the base upon which many disorders are expressed in the body.

The internal Organs—Liver, Spleen, Heart, Lung, and Kidney—are the material base for Emotions, the place where they take root.

Emotions may provoke disorders in the internal Organs. Likewise, dysfunctions of the internal Organs can affect the mind, conditioning it to manifest Emotions corresponding to the imbalanced Organ.

In the words of Ricardo Fernández Herrero, when an Organ is affected, it releases into the mind the predisposition to feel a determined Emotion.

We mentioned already in the previous chapter that the influence of the internal Organs is seen in different areas of the body—sensory Organs, tissues, body fluids—and also in the emotional and psychological spheres. This influence can be explained, in part, by the Five Movements with which they correspond as well as the physiological functions and channels (meridians) related to each Organ. Once again, we see evidence of Chinese Medicine's conception of the human being as an integrated whole.

Emotions are not only one of the causes of illness, but can also be observed as symptoms in various syndromes related to the Organs, to Blood, and to Energy.

When referring to Emotions as a cause of illness, they are referred to as the Seven Sentiments or Seven Passions. These are Anger, Excitement or Joy, Sadness, Grief, Worry, Fear, and Fright or Terror.

As we've seen in table 2.1, Emotions are also associated with the

Five Movements. Wood is associated with Anger, Fire with Joy, Earth with Worry, Metal with Sadness, and Water with Fear.

In order to better understand Emotions and how Chinese Medicine views them, and before commenting on them one by one, I'd like to highlight a few aspects that may be of interest to us.

- Each one of the Emotions affects Energy in a particular way, compelling it to behave in a certain manner. The Flower Remedies, by modifying emotional states, influence Energy. We'll see how to put this knowledge into practice.
- Also, all Emotions affect the Heart, which coordinates the functioning of the Organs and Viscera. When disturbed, all functions are influenced and become imbalanced.
- The Organs most disturbed by imbalanced emotional activity are the Heart, Spleen, and Liver.
- We should also be aware that the relationship between an Emotion and an Organ is not static but rather is a tool that can help orient us when working with clients. Emotions really affect the whole body. The whole body is conscious, and as we've come to see, its parts are all interrelated: Organs, tissues, Emotions.

Anger

When impetus and assertion (aspects of the Liver's Psyche, explained in the next chapter) are hindered or become imbalanced, anger arises.

When the impulse that carries us forward and gives us the ability to face obstacles becomes unsuccessful, barriers seem formidable or we just don't have the strength to move through difficulties. It's something like when a child can't get his toy to work and finally throws it against the wall, enraged. Which is why anger carries with it a certain degree of frustration when it's related with what we've just stated above. It accompanies indignation, and it rises up against injustice.

Some people get all up in arms when even the smallest thing goes wrong. It is also true that anger is an Emotion that impels, and we've all seen people who use it as a means of transport, as a way to initiate action and do things.

Another aspect of this Emotion is its usefulness with regard to danger; it allows us to react. It is a survival tool that helps to manifest Water (fear), which feels danger. Anger helps us react as a consequence, so we can see why anger is very often one of the faces of fear. Notice the link between the Movement of Water and the Movement of Wood, according to the Generating Cycle.

We find people who are in a constant state of alert because they feel danger in every situation. This in itself can be a cause of insomnia.

We can also see that anger has to do with self-affirmation, with "here I am," affirming individuality. Imbalanced anger is an Emotion that separates. It interrupts like Wind does, snatching up everything and tossing it around. Expressed out of harmony, it implies the need to affirm oneself in opposition to someone else.

Expressions of Anger

Expressions of anger include resentment, contained rage, irritability, annoyance, vexation, frustration, animosity, bitterness, and feeling offended.

The Movement of Energy and the Organ Affected

- It makes Energy ascend.
- It affects the Liver.

Symptoms

Symptoms are manifested in the upper part of the body.

In the head and neck: headache, migraine, ringing in the ears, red splotches at the front of the neck, reddened face, thirst, red tongue, bitter taste in the mouth.

Serious cases may present fainting and stroke. A common symptom is recurring migraines. There may even be diarrhea and vomiting of blood.

Liver Blood and Liver yin influence in the predisposition to feel anger. Deficiencies in Liver Blood and Liver yin tend to make a person cantankerous or even explosive.

When the Emotion persists over time or is very intense, it can disturb functioning of the Stomach, Spleen, and Kidney, generating symptoms that will lead us to investigate anger in the person.

These may be expressions when the following Organs are affected:

- Stomach: hiccups, belches, vomiting
- Spleen: abdominal distention, diarrhea with undigested food
- Kidney: memory loss, fear, debility of lumbar vertebrae, weakened knees

This is an Emotion that may be masking many others like depression, fear, or shame. Anger is generally more socially accepted than other Emotions it could be covering.

When anger continues but is no longer expressed—when the flow begins to fade away—resentment begins to appear, and the person starts showing behavior that is aggressive at its base.

If the person reaches a point of true balance regarding this Emotion, he has the capacity to exercise it with a great gentleness.

Joy

Feeling the expansiveness of life gives birth to a kind of joy closer to serenity than the kind of agitated, almost euphoric joy so common these days.

It is a kind of joy whose Fire doesn't oblige one to lose the calmness that Metal provides; it doesn't toss serenity and clarity out of the Heart.

When joy is not insistently accompanied by constant stimulus and sought as the only Emotion to be had—which is to say, when it is spontaneous—it fortifies health. It distends and relaxes. It improves all the Organs' functioning and favors a smooth flow of Blood, Energy, and fluids.

Expressions of Joy
Joy also refers to excitability, need for stimulus, hyperemotiveness, and boisterous laughter.

Movement of Energy and Organ Affected
- It relaxes Energy.
- It affects the Heart.

In ancient texts like the *Su Wen* (which forms part of the *Huang Di Nei Jing*), it's been written that joy is a very beneficial Emotion. If it is experienced harmoniously—most of all when it's not forced, as occurs in Agrimony states—it favors the Heart's proper functioning. Nutritive Energy and Defensive Energy (which are explained in chapter 4) flow in harmony.

Joy has a balancing effect, making Energy more harmonious and favoring a relaxed and peaceful state of mind.

The problem arises when joy becomes excessive. It tends to disperse Energy, especially that of the Heart, so *Shen*, who lives there, loses his place of residence, generating various disorders (see chapter 6, "The Psyches").

Symptoms

Symptoms usually seen in joy-related imbalances are:

- Palpitations, laughter and crying, restlessness, much talk, alternating euphoria and depression
- Insomnia, reduced memory, difficulties in concentrating, mental weariness

When joy is exaggerated and insistent, the road leads to bitterness.

Sadness

According to some authors, sadness is related to compassion—the capacity to feel the suffering of others and to register it as sorrow.

It somehow allows us to unite with others, to be capable of getting out of ourselves and to perceive pain, even when it isn't our own.

It is the Emotion of that which is ending, of the separation from that which is beloved to us. And if we view it in terms of the annual cycle, it is the sadness of the end of summer and the beginning of autumn. Plenitude has passed and the season of loss has arrived.

In our society, which doesn't want to have anything to do with the ending of things, there isn't much space for sadness; it is tolerated for a little while and then—time to get those bells back on your toes. Activity and joy are overvalued.

Sadness also implies a sentiment preceding it, signifying its balanced expression: a withdrawal for reflection. The time for action has passed (which isn't to say that it won't return), and from a place of serenity, of quieting down, we begin to gather Energy into ourselves for reflection and evaluation.

On the other hand, when sadness is plainly out of balance, it becomes disdain, indifference, and a critical attitude. The person becomes increasingly more critical. Notice how the sentiment and its function have become perversed, moving from evaluation and reflection to critique.

Expressions of Sadness

Sadness includes suffering, sorrow, grief, melancholy, unhappiness, anxiety, and pessimism.

Movement of Energy and Organ Affected

• It diminishes and dissolves Energy.
• It affects the Lung.

In influencing the Lung—and through it, Energy—sadness takes away our strength and willpower. The Lung helps us obtain Energy from the air. When its functioning is altered due to sadness, one of the sources of Energy is reduced, and we become debilitated; our capacity for action dwindles, and it becomes difficult to remedy this state without help. The Flower Remedies are obviously of almost unequivocal value and utility in these cases.

Symptoms

Associated symptoms are short and shallow breathing, faint voice, cough, general weakness, depressed body and temperament, weakened will, laziness, sighs, thoracic oppression, crying, weariness.

Sadness in women can upset the menstrual cycle, generating amenorrhea (absence of menstruation). It also influences the Blood, generating deficiencies.

If this Emotion impacts the Heart, we may see palpitations and reduced concentration.

If it impacts the Liver, there may be pain and spasms in the ribs, tight muscles, and possibly eye troubles.

If it affects the Spleen, weakness of the limbs, abdominal distention, and/or diarrhea with undigested food may result.

Grief

This Emotion generates disturbances similar to those of sadness.

Movement of Energy and Organ Affected
• It diminishes Energy.
• It disturbs the Lung.

Symptoms
Symptoms that may be observed are Energy deficiency and despondency. The person cries easily, and his enthusiasm and capacity for undertaking projects is notably reduced. Likewise, as Eric Marié writes in his book *Compendio de Medicina China* (Summary of Chinese Medicine), clarity of Spirit is disturbed.

Worry

Reflection, which is the balanced Emotion of the Spleen, and thought are necessary capacities we humans possess. They allow us to take available information, analyze it, and organize it in order to resolve situations.

When these are out of balance, worry arises. Uncertainty favors this Emotion.

Expressions of Worry
Expressions of worry include reflection, obsession, excessive thought, and rumination.

Movement of Energy and Organ Affected
• It stagnates Energy.
• It affects the Spleen.

Excessive studying, too much thinking, and doing too much mental-related work debilitate the Spleen, influencing the Heart and its Blood.

Symptoms

Symptoms of worry may be weariness, a bland disposition, lack of appetite, chest and abdominal distention, vertigo, insomnia or disturbed sleep, palpitations, forgetfulness, mental fatigue, and weight loss. As the Spleen loses its functional capacity, phlegm and mucus may accumulate in the body, and the Lung is one of its depositories.

Giovanni Maciocia in his book, *The Foundations of Chinese Medicine,* tells us that worry disturbs the Lung's activity, generating anxiety, shallow breathing, and tension in the shoulders and neck. He says, "The shallow and short breathing of a person who is sad and worried is an expression of the constraint of the corporal soul and Lung-Qi."

He notes that many people show tense, hunched-up shoulders with shallow breathing, typical of blocked Lung Energy due to chronic worry.

If the worrying is particularly chronic, it can generate a feeling of aversion, of not wanting more of anything. The person may find it hard to feel gratitude.

Nostalgia

Nostalgia knots up Energy, disturbing digestion, with symptoms similar to those of worry. It can also harm Heart-Blood, with symptoms such as insomnia, palpitations, disturbed sleep, and vertigo.

Fear

Fear clearly keeps us alive when we're in danger by keeping us alert. Then again, it can restrict life to such an extent that it paralyzes and ultimately drowns a person.

Chronic fear can mutate into paranoia and lead the person to overvalue secrecy and to live in secrecy. As we can see, it's another form of restraint.

Expressions of Fear

Expressions of fear include phobia, panic, apprehension, and cowardice.

Movement of Energy and Organ Affected

- It makes Energy descend.
- It affects the Kidney.

Symptoms

The Energy spent when this Emotion is out of balance comes from the Kidney.

Energy descends, showing symptoms such as weakness in the knees, shaking of the knees, and fecal and urinary incontinence if the Energy descends abruptly. When urination is frequent and tends to be transparent, after ruling out other disorders, it would be wise to investigate possible fears.

Kidney Energy, when it is weak, generates states of fear. The same occurs when Blood and Energy are deficient.

The Gallbladder is a special Viscera; it's not just a Viscera. It governs determination and decision and is related to courage and audacity. When this Viscera is weak, it favors a lack of courage and bravery. And there we have its relationship with fear.

Terror

Expressions of Terror

Among expressions of terror are fright, panic, and shock.

Movement of Energy and Organ Affected

- It disorganizes Energy.
- It affects the Heart and the Kidney.

The Heart is affected suddenly, reducing its Energy.

Symptoms

Frequent symptoms are palpitations, shallow and short breathing, nervousness, mental confusion, loss of breath, fainting, and insomnia.

The Kidney is disrupted because its Essence must be used to supplement the sudden drop in Energy. This sudden shock can cause night sweats, dryness of the mouth, vertigo, and ringing in the ears.

The Five Emotions
May Be Transformed into Fire

When Emotions are persistent or strong, they generate Energy stagnation, which, when long-standing, produces Fire.

Some symptoms may be insomnia, a bitter taste in the mouth, irritability, and dark urine. It can be helpful to look at the person's tongue as it may be red, dry, and sometimes red at the tip. The other symptoms will depend on the Organ affected.

Working with the Flowers and Emotions

So, there are a variety of points to make:

- Knowing the effect that each Emotion has on Energy allows us to choose Flowers to help balance this effect. For example, if the person consulting with us tells us that, among other Emotions, **sadness** is the most frequent or most present at that moment, then we, knowing how sadness acts on Energy, can help the action of the Flowers we've chosen by adding those that favor an increase in Energy. We might add Olive, Hornbeam, Clematis, Oak, Centaury—whichever is most appropriate for the person in question. Also, we would evaluate which of the Flowers that act on obsession—and any others that act on the Spleen—would be pertinent for that person. The Spleen is another Organ that generates Blood and Energy. If we help regulate Emotions affecting it, we favor the production of Energy. In regulating sadness, we are treating the cause of the person's Energy loss (though there may be other causes). In modulating the Emotions that disturb the Spleen, we are trying to maintain the Energy that this Organ provides, which will help the action of Flowers like Mustard.
- Knowing which is the most powerful Emotion or Emotions in the person consulting us, we can investigate the possible presence of the physical and/or emotional symptoms that accompany that Emotion. During follow-up visits, we'll keep these symptoms in mind with the intention of preventing them and observing their evolution.
- Understanding that Emotions generate specific physical effects in the body and are accompanied by other psychological and emotional

symptoms, we can conceive (from the Chinese Medicine point of how the Flowers act on physical symptoms. They do so thr relationship that the Flower-related Emotion has with the symptoms. For example, we can understand why it is that Holly diminishes or eliminates dizziness, headaches, and a bitter taste in the mouth.

- Knowledge from Chinese Medicine can be a great resource to us in that it allows us to deduce Emotions based on physical symptoms. It's not about trying to theorize and seeing what happens; our deduction comes from conclusions based on thousands of years of observation. Although we won't use this knowledge perfectly, nor use it automatically, it *is* reliable information. We can use this knowledge to discover Emotions that the patient is unaware of and this discovery can in itself be therapeutic. It's not unusual to receive consultations from people who would like to be treated with Flower Essences but who don't tell us about one single Emotion.

- We can use Flower Essences to treat the emotional and physical symptoms that arise as a consequence of a base Emotion. Let's clarify this statement: we'll consider the Emotion that we're treating, for example, fear, as the cause of the disorders it provokes. Then there are symptoms, which are the product of the imbalance, also needing treatment.

- A word about obsessions: discovering together with our clients which of their obsessions are the most powerful and, if possible, the most long-standing, we'll be in a position to heal one of the most important ways in which Energy is drained. I'm not only talking about obsessions expressed as thoughts (although they equally drain Energy) but also those that end up manifesting themselves in actions. Helping to regulate these aspects, though not entirely easy, not only frees the person but also puts more Energy at her disposal so that the body can repair itself and the person can better approach the changes she needs to make happen.

- When dealing with **anger**, Holly is appropriate, not only because it regulates the Emotion but also because it favors the descent of Energy. Elm can support Holly, to help contain the overflow of ascending Energy characteristic of this Emotion. We would normally choose Cherry Plum without even knowing about Chinese Medicine, but we'd also use it from the Chinese Medicine point of view, as Energy tends to ascend in an uncontrolled manner.

This Emotion usually generates Heat and inflammation, which can be treated with Holly; it's equally wise to use Vervain, as it helps to settle Heat and inflammation, as well as to treat irradiation that, in anger, is directed upward.

Another essence that can lighten our work with this Emotion is Clematis, which helps keep a person grounded, counterbalancing the ascension of Energy. Also, anger produces disconnection, treatable with Clematis.

At the moment, we use Water Violet and Rock Water when Blood and yin need support. While we continue observing the effects of other, more specific, options, these Flowers have demonstrated their beneficial effects often enough that we use them to this end.

Blood and yin have close relationships with body fluids. Walnut helps avoid the loss of fluids—and of Blood in hemorrhages—thus avoiding Blood and yin deficiencies.

Cherry Plum also helps with fluids. When there is too much control, it is not unusual that in some other area the same person is out of control. We've seen, in some people, excessive elimination of fluids: this is how they express their lack of control. It's also necessary to clarify that in other people Cherry Plum favors the elimination of those liquids that had been controlled with an iron fist before taking the essence.

- In reference to **joy**, Cerato is a Flower that helps to regulate the Energy dispersal generated by imbalances related to this Emotion. Hornbeam helps in the sense that it regulates the excessive lassitude that occurs after an "acute attack" of joy. It restores tone.

  It's possible to go as far as a Wild Rose state after the overexcitement and excessive stimulus, and let's not forget Olive.

  Scleranthus (due to alternating symptoms) and Impatiens (once again we see acceleration) can help regulate some of the symptoms that are products of imbalances in joy. Heather helps with the excessive verbalization. Persons in Heather and Agrimony states can fall into frankly cacophonous states of joy.

- We can work on **worry** with essences that remove obstructions, and these essences will likewise help work on whichever obsession or fixation presents itself. Crab Apple, Chicory, Willow (which also favor the dissolution of mucus), Red Chestnut, and Heather are indicated

Flowers. Honeysuckle, in states of worry and obsession and even in reflective states, is always moving backward. Chestnut Bud is useful in rumination, and White Chestnut is also indicated, for the element of repetition.

It would also be wise to support Energy in the presence of these Emotions, given that the Spleen's Energy production is affected. We can do so with Olive, Centaury, Clematis, Hornbeam, and others.

For **nostalgia**, Honeysuckle's action is evident, but Flowers suggested for worry and its family of Emotions are also useful.

- When dealing with **fear**, Mimulus not only treats a type of fear but also prevents Energy from being drained downward. Mustard and Gentian are currently being tested for their ability to regulate the descent of Energy.

Rock Rose can modulate the disorganization of Energy generated by terror and fright.

It's wise to help the Gallbladder when fear is an issue, and we can do so with Centaury and Willow. We'll also want to nourish Energy with the Flowers mentioned above, Olive being especially applicable due to its relationship with the Kidney.

4

Energy and Blood

Energy

*T*he concept of Energy takes us back to the ancient Chinese world-view, according to which all that exists in the universe is formed by it.

Each time we wish to define some component of the Chinese grand scheme, including Chinese Medicine theory, we find ourselves facing dilemmas difficult to resolve.

In the case of Energy, its very nature of impulse, movement, transformation, and change make the task of defining it look something like trying to catch a gust of wind with a butterfly net. Energy is also insubstantial compared to other more solid aspects, like Blood.

Wang Fu Zhi (1619–1692), quoted in Giovanni Maciocia's *The Foundations of Chinese Medicine*, expressed it in this way: "All that is void and empty is full of Qi which, in its state of condensation and thus visible, is called being, but in its state of dispersion and thus no longer visible, is called nonbeing," and "when dispersing Qi makes the Great Void, only regaining its original misty form but not perishing; when condensing it becomes the origin of all beings."

It might be more interesting to approach the Chinese Medicine grand scheme as if it were a game that goes about leaving us clues. When we arrive at the place indicated by one of the clues, we find more clues leading us to other places. The journey and the movement from one place to the next gives us a better idea about the subjects we're trying to understand than does a simple photograph of just one aspect without its relationship to other aspects. Continuing with our attempt to understand something about Energy, we could say that it is a bit Ceratic:* it is itself, but it adopts different faces and names according to the function it fulfills, the place where it appears, and how it originates.

For example, if we focus on the Liver, Energy takes on characteristics related to the Organ's functions, in this case making sure that everything in the body circulates at a constant rhythm, without obstructions or stagnation. But if we refer to Defensive Energy, we see that it carries out the function of protecting the organism from pathogens like Wind, Cold, Dampness, and so on.

Regarding the translation of the Chinese expression *Qi,* the word most often used is *Energy,* although we can find others like breath, vital force, vapor.

We find the origin of Energy in the interaction between yin and yang, which generates Movement, activity, change, growth, and development.

Functions of Energy

Warming

Energy maintains body temperature, favoring the circulation of Blood and organic fluids. At the right temperature, Blood flows freely. When Blood is affected by Cold, it stagnates.

Warming also promotes the evaporation of organic fluids, and this is another way to avoid stagnation.

Energy deficiency generates disorders in the function of warming, producing the following symptoms: aversion to cold, chilly lumbar area, reduced body temperature, cold extremities, stagnation of Blood and fluids, and disorders in Blood production.

Impulse

Energy impels the growth and development of the organism.

Impulse also favors the functioning of the Organs and Viscera, as

---

*[Referring to the Cerato Flower Essence. —*Trans.*]

well as that of the meridians. This aspect of Energy actively participates in the production and circulation of Blood and organic fluids.

When impulse is weak, the activity of vital Organs, tissues, and meridians is reduced. The production of Blood and organic fluids is affected, and their circulation is slowed, causing Blood deficiency or fluid retention. In serious cases, the growth and development of the organism may be affected, possibly even resulting in early senility. Various occurrences of hypofunctioning may be observed, as well as disturbances in the elimination of waste products.

Transformation

Blood, Essence, organic fluids, and Energy are all subject to uninterrupted transformations. All body functions depend on this activity.

For example, food is transformed into nutritive substances, Qi, Blood, organic fluids, and Essence. After being metabolized, they transform into sweat, urine, nasal discharge, saliva; in other words, waste products. After digestion and absorption, food residue is also converted into waste products that are eliminated from the body.

Inefficacy of this function produces problems in digestion and assimilation of nutrients, in the production of vital substances, and in the transformation and elimination of waste products.

Control

Energy checks and controls Essence, Blood, and body fluids, preventing them from escaping in nonphysiological ways. This includes maintaining the Viscera in place, preventing gravity from changing their position.

The Spleen's Energy keeps Blood in the veins and arteries in this manner, and the Kidney's Energy controls the lower orifices.

This function of Energy is also expressed in the maintenance of the fetus by placing it in its usual position, avoiding disturbances, and favoring its normal development.

When control is weak, Blood leaks out, and there may be hemorrhaging and loss of fluids through perspiration, urinary incontinence, excess salivation, nocturnal emissions (spermatorrhoea), miscarriages, and premature labor.

Protection

Energy defends us from the penetration of external pathogenic factors and fights against them when they are found present in the body.

When there is a deficiency in this aspect, diminished immune capacity occurs, and one is much more vulnerable to external Energies. As this protective Energy lacks adequate potency for fighting against said factors, illnesses last longer and relapses occur more frequently.

Origin of Energy

Innate Essence: passed down from parents.
Acquired Essence: subtle Essence from food and air.

Production of Energy

Related with the following Organs:

* Kidney stores innate Essence.
* Stomach and Spleen produce acquired Essence.
* Lung obtains Energy from air and is master and distributor of Energy.

Let's look at an example of a very simple application for the Flowers.

Knowing that the Kidney, Spleen, and Lung are fundamental in the production of Energy, it is very important to regulate the Emotions and Psyches, which, when out of balance, could affect these Organs.

We'll perceive which of the Emotions related with these three Organs are most present in the person consulting us, and we'll use the corresponding Flowers.

For example, a person in a White Chestnut state and with a tendency toward Elm will exhibit altered functioning of the Spleen and, consequently, a reduced production of Blood and Energy.

Different Types of Energy

Essence

Essence is the force that creates and sustains the human body. The part that we receive directly from our parents we call innate Essence. The other part, coming from Energy from the air, foods, and liquids we breathe, eat, and drink, we call acquired Essence. It is the subtle

Essence we take in from these sources that forms acquired Essence. It complements and supports innate Essence.

Original Energy

Original Energy comes from innate Essence supported by acquired Essence. It is manufactured in the Kidney.

Fundamental Energy

Fundamental Energy is produced out of Energy from the air, brought in by the Lung, and Energy from food, distilled in the Spleen.

Nutritive Energy

Energy obtained from the transformation of food is carried by the Spleen toward the Lung; the most refined part goes to the blood vessels and channels (meridians) to be circulated with Blood and Energy as Nutritive Energy.

Defensive Energy

This Energy is also extracted from food by the Spleen. When the Spleen transports it to the Lung, the most subtle part leaves the meridians and constitutes Defensive Energy. This Energy is very light and mobile and is so subtle that it can't be contained by the meridians. It's the Energy that protects us from external pathogenic factors like Wind and Cold.

Blood

Blood and Energy are indissolubly associated. We can think of Blood as a more material manifestation of Energy, like a more dense Energy. Without Energy, Blood would be a lifeless fluid and therefore lack the vital importance it possesses.

Nevertheless, Blood is objectively material; it's the red fluid that circulates through the veins and arteries, a very nutritive fluid, one of the most vitally basic components of the human body. It circulates through the blood vessels which are "Blood's residence." Eric Marié tells us, in his book *Compendio de Medicina China,* that the ideogram depicts "a ritual recipient full of Blood, that is used for the occasion of a ceremonial offering."

Production

The nutritive substances transformed from food and liquids (absorption and digestion) by the Spleen and Stomach are the material base for the formation of Blood.

The Essence from food ascends to the Lung and Heart and there is transformed into Blood through the function of the transformation of Energy.

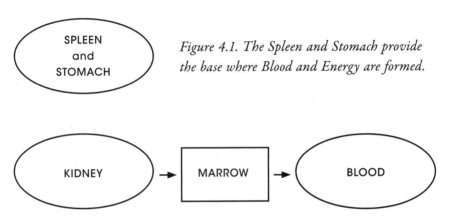

Figure 4.1. The Spleen and Stomach provide the base where Blood and Energy are formed.

Figure 4.2. The Kidney stores the Essence from which marrow is made, which in turn makes Blood.

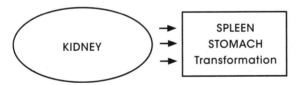

Figure 4.3. Kidney Energy also helps the Spleen and Stomach in their functions of transformation and transport of food.

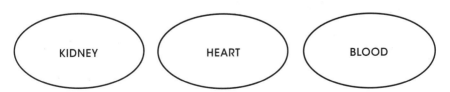

Figure 4.4. Kidney Energy also helps the Heart and Lungs in their functions of Blood distribution.

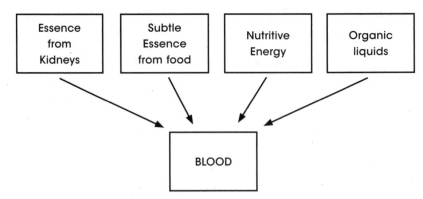

Figure 4.5. Blood is made of Nutritive Energy,
organic fluids, and Kidney Essence.

How Blood Circulates

Blood moves through the body without interruption thanks to the impulse provided by Energy, expressed as the joint action of the Organs.

The Heart, Lung, Liver, and Spleen participate.

- The **Heart** provides the initial impulse and pushes the Blood.
- The **Lung** distributes Blood to the entire body.
- The **Liver** stores Blood; it is its reservoir and regulates it by sending it to different parts of the body as needed. It manages the volume of Blood in the organism.
- The **Spleen** prevents Blood from flowing over and leaking out.

It is important that the blood vessels are in good condition, and this depends on the condition of the Heart's Energy and its Blood. Also:

> The Liver fluidifies blood.
> The Lung cleans and enriches it.
> The Kidney and Lung clean it.

Blood's Functions

Nourishes and Moistens

Blood nourishes the whole organism, while also moistening all the areas through which it circulates. When, for a variety of reasons, this function is deficient, the following symptoms may be observed:

- Dry skin
- Tense muscles
- General weakness
- Reduced rhythm of the functional activity of the Viscera

The Material Base for Mental and Spiritual Activity
Insufficiency or dysfunction of the Blood influences the neurological, mental, and emotional spheres. The following symptoms may be produced when disorders are present:

- Insomnia
- Memory loss
- Agitation
- Loss of consciousness
- Psychiatric disorders
- Coma

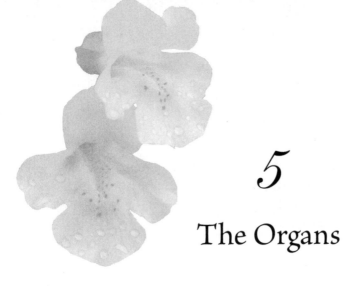

5

The Organs

*E*ven if this is just going to be a quick overview, we do need to know some fundamental ideas regarding Chinese Medicine's conception of the Organs.

In Chinese Medicine, the concept of Organ does not only cover its tissue and functions but also implies a vast range of actions including various other tissues, sensory Organs, fluids, and orifices, as well as a clear influence in the emotional, psychological, and spiritual realms.

Clearly, just as an Organ's functioning determines in part one's emotional and psychological state, Emotions, thoughts, sensations, and spiritual states powerfully influence the harmony and functioning of the Organs.

This view of the Organs lets us understand the importance, regarding our health, of methods for quieting the mind, as they help us to maintain a balanced state. Quieting the mind is probably one of the most effective forms of preventing and curing imbalances. We tend to identify ourselves with our mind and its contents (Emotions and thoughts, for example), believing that these are all that we are. We live inside our heads, in a symbolic construction of the world, and we inhabit our bodies very little in the sense of perceiving our sensations without interpreting them. We forget that the whole body is conscious (as stated in chapter 3, about the Emotions) and that we learn through the totality of who we are, including every little body part.

As Gabriel Nieto, director of Escuela Taoísta del Sur (South Daoist School), says, "Don't pay too much attention to the radio in the room [the mind constantly transmitting thoughts, sentiments, and so on]; just go about your business, the radio is not that important."

One way to regulate the mind—to pay it less attention and reconnect the many fragmented parts of ourselves—is through the Flowers. The Flowers are an immensely valuable tool when the mind needs adjusting and quieting in order to focus on the present moment and the lesson that is at hand. Bach himself mentions many times in his writings the importance of retreating to a quiet place with a still mind in order to hear the soul's mandates. He states, "Doctrines and civilisation have robbed us of Silence, have robbed us of the Knowledge that WE KNOW ALL WITHIN OURSELVES" (Howard and Ramsell, *The Original Writings of Edward Bach*, 136).

Moreover, in this day and age, replete with various methods for balancing ourselves, for having more Energy, living longer, having a higher sexual capacity, and more resistance, we easily lose sight of the reason for gaining all this. If we achieve a higher Energy level, what do we want to use it for? Do we know our own true path? It is very common to dilapidate this increased Energy level, which we so obsessively achieved, by being just the same as we ever were and messing up with more vigor.

Reining ourselves back in from this tangent, let's return to the Organs and take a look at more relationships that can help us both in our work with the Flowers and in finding our own balance.

The Five Organs

When we speak of the Organs in Chinese Medicine, we are referring to the theory of the *Zang Fu* (Organs and Viscera). So let's take this opportunity to talk about the Organs as they serve as a very important bridge between the Emotions, Psyches, and body.

The Five Organs are Liver, Heart, Spleen, Lung, and Kidney. These are five systems, interrelated and in communication with the entire organism via the meridians (Energy's circulatory pathways), which unite internal with external, up with down, one side with the other. The physiological relationships between the Organs can be explained based on the Five Movements.

The Organs are the center of a web of correspondences and extend their influence to the tissues and regions of the body that they nourish and impregnate with their characteristics.

Their functions are to produce, transform, conserve, and store valuable substances that are essential to life. They are the material base of the various psychological, emotional, and spiritual expressions.

This concept integrates the emotional and psychological world with the totality of the person, including the body. The Organs' areas of influence can be affected by Emotions, and this provides us with a map that reveals the paths of the Emotions in the body.

The Organs store pure substances previously refined by the Viscera. They store Energy, Blood, organic fluids, and Essence (coming from the Energy we receive from our parents plus that which we obtain from food and air).

When the Organs are functioning well, it is possible to inhabit the body, to be incarnate, to have consciousness present in matter.

At the same time, they influence the capacity to carry out the inverse trajectory, from the corporal and material to the subtle. They allow us to refine and to nourish ourselves from that which is pure and transformed.

The Spirit roots itself in the Organs. There, it purifies, refines, and makes substance lighter, and we likewise find there the capacity for making things concrete and material, without losing sight of the more subtle aspects of the world.

Each Organ houses a type of Spirit, which in Chinese Medicine is called the Visceral Spirits. They are also called the Psyches, and this is how we will refer to them. We will develop the Psyches as a topic in the next chapter.

Flower Essences, by adjusting emotional and psychological aspects, influence the entire range of the Organs' actions, thus opening possibilities for prevention and healing. And as we've already pointed out in other parts of this book, it is also possible, from the Chinese Medicine viewpoint, to explain how the Flowers affect various parts of the body.

Physiological Functions of the Organs

We will comment on each Organ's functions and the symptoms that are generated when not functioning adequately.

Each time there is a reference to the term *Qi,* we are referring to Energy.

Liver Organ

Location	Right side of upper abdomen (right hypochondrium)
Element with which it relates	Wood
Hours	1 a.m. to 3 a.m.
Season	Spring
Time of day	Dawn
Associated Viscera	Gallbladder

Physiological Functions

Drainage and Dispersion

- Enables the free flow of Qi, balancing Qi's mechanism, harmony of the functional activity of the Viscera
- Regulates Emotions
- Stimulates digestion and food assimilation by supporting the Spleen's and Stomach's ascending and descending Movements
- Produces bile
- Averts stagnation of Blood, Energy, and organic fluids
- Maintains regularity of *Chong Mai* and *Ren Mai* (two of the Extraordinary Meridians, the first related to Blood and the second to the body's yin)

Blood Storage

- It retains a quantity of Blood, which nourishes it and controls Liver yang.
- It nourishes tendons and eyes.
- It regulates Chong Mai and prevents uterine hemorrhages.
- It regulates the amount of Blood that goes to various body parts according to activity (varies according to exertion, Emotions).
- When at rest, this Blood returns to the Liver.

Dysfunctions

Disorders in Drainage and Dispersion

Stagnation of Energy Circulation
- Irritability, orneriness, depression, worry, mistrust, suspicion
- Pain and distension in chest, hypochondrium (upper abdominal region), breasts, sides of abdomen, groin
- Lack of appetite, belching, vomiting, diarrhea, abdominal distension
- Occasionally, jaundice
- Pain in various parts of the body

Stagnation of Blood Circulation
- Pinching pain
- Menstrual disorders like amenorrhea, dysmenorrhea, coagulated Blood
- Gynecological tumors with a defined shape, pain, and sensitivity

Prolonged Stagnation Generates Fire
- Seriously hot tempered
- Headaches and vertigo
- Ringing in the ears, hearing problems, red eyes
- Insomnia, sleep disorders

Fire Becomes Wind
- Vertigo
- Tremors
- Convulsions

Disorders in Storing Blood
- Paleness
- Dry eyes, blurred vision, diminished night vision
- Tendon and muscle spasms
- Numbness in the extremities, difficulty moving
- Light menstrual flow, long cycle, absence of menstruation
- Abundant menstruation, uterine hemorrhaging

Body Regions

- Eyes
- Fingernails and toenails
- Tendons
- Tears

Disorders

- Eyes: congestion, diminished night vision, blurred vision, dry eyes, reduced vision, strabismus (crossed eyes), glaring, tearing, myopia, tendency to contract infectious conjunctivitis, allergies, yellow secretions
- Nails: split, discolored, dull, dry, soft, deformed
- Tendons: tremors, spasms in the extremities

Heart Organ

Location	Thoracic cavity
Element with which it relates	Fire
Hours	11 a.m. to 1 p.m.
Season	Summer
Time of day	Midday
Associated Viscera	Small intestine

Physiological Functions

Controls Blood and Vessels

- Where Qi from food is transformed into Blood
- Pumps Blood
- Condition of blood vessels depends upon the Heart's Blood and Qi

Governs Mental and Spiritual Activity

- Vitality; expresses the general coherency of the organism's functions
- Psychological and spiritual aspects
- Organizing consciousness that expresses itself through the Visceral Spirits
- General harmony of the Viscera depends upon Shen (for more on Shen, see chapter 6, "The Psyches")

Dysfunctions

Disorders in Controlling Blood and Vessels
- Cold hands
- Fatigue
- Feeble physical constitution, little strength

Heart Energy Deficiency
- Pale face, pale tongue
- Shortness of breath
- Heart palpitations, occasionally arrhythmia

Blood Stagnation
- Purplish face, tongue (possibly with purple splotches), and lips
- Chest pain, or pain beneath the sternum
- Piercing pain

Heart Blood Deficiency
- Pale cast to the skin
- Pale tongue
- Palpitations
- Vertigo

Disorders in Governing Mental and Spiritual Activity
- Absentminded, distracted
- Unclear thinking
- Poor memory
- Depression
- Anxiety
- Mental restlessness
- Daytime agitation and palpitations
- Insomnia and sleep disturbances
- Laziness
- Delirium; in severe cases, loss of consciousness

Body Regions
- Face
- Blood vessels

- Sweat
- Tongue

Disorders
- Face: pale, red, purplish
- Tongue: pale, purplish, difficulty speaking, stiffness, aphasia
- Blood vessels: imbalances in Blood circulation
- Sweat: scarce or abundant, sweating with minimal effort or Emotion, copious and cold, night sweats

Spleen Organ

Location	Upper left abdomen (left hypochondrium)
Element with which it relates	Earth
Hours	9 a.m. to 11 a.m.
Season	Between Summer and Fall
Time of day	Afternoon
Associated Viscera	Stomach

Physiological Functions

Transport and Transformation
- Digestion and metabolism.
- Extracts the subtle Essence from food and drink that it receives from the Stomach and transports it to the whole organism for nourishing tissues. This function has two aspects:

  1. In relation to solid food and drink, which will make up Blood's base, Defensive Energy and acquired *Jing* (Essence)
  2. In relation to fluids—transporting and transforming water and Dampness

Ascent of That Which Is Pure
- Subtle Essence from foods is transported toward the Lung.
- The Spleen's ascending Energy sustains the whole of the Viscera, preventing them from distending and dropping.

Blood Production and Control
- Participates in Blood production due to its function of transformation.
- Keeps Blood inside the blood vessels.

Dysfunctions

Disorders in Transporting and Transforming
- Apathy
- Poor digestion
- Reduced appetite, abdominal distension
- Soft stools, diarrhea, weight loss
- Weariness, weakness, shallow breathing
- Paleness
- Edema, mucus (chest feels full, nausea, vomiting, cough, asthma)
- Obesity

Disorders in Ascending That Which Is Pure

Reduced Production of Blood and Energy
- Fainting, vertigo, blurred vision
- Weariness
- Chronic diarrhea
- Abundant menstruation
- Prolapsed Stomach, Kidney, uterus, anus; hernias

Disorders in Producing and Controlling Blood
- Pale face
- Insomnia
- Vertigo, fainting
- Hemorrhaging, uterine bleeding, hematuria, spontaneous bruising, Blood in feces

Body Regions
- Mouth, lips
- Saliva
- Muscles, limbs

Disorders
- Mouth: anomalies in flavor perception, pasty mouth, sugary flavor
- Lips: pale, dry, dull, cracked lips
- Saliva: excess salivation
- Muscles: weakness, atrophy, cold, weariness in the limbs, weight loss

Lung Organ

Location	Thorax
Element with which it relates	Metal
Hours	3 a.m. to 5 a.m.
Season	Autumn
Time of day	Sunset
Associated Viscera	Large Intestine

Physiological Functions

Governs Energy
- Governs breath (respiratory Energy) and the whole body's Qi
- Captures part of external Energy that comes with breath
- Receives food Energy that has been metabolized by the Spleen and Stomach: *Zhong Qi* (ensuring breathing and cardiac functioning) is thus formed
- Governs Energy circulation and has an important role in balancing ascending and descending Movements as well as internalization and externalization
- Influences the Movements of Blood and body fluids

Governs Diffusion, Descent, and Purification
- Qi and body fluids (toward the Kidney)
- Purification: the Lung's eliminatory function
- Through its functions of diffusion, descent, and purification

Dysfunctions

Disorders in Governing Energy
- Dyspnea, chest discomfort
- Shallow breathing, asthma

- Weak voice
- Weariness
- Diminished Defensive Energy

Disorders in Diffusing, Descending, and Purifying
- Cough, asthma, dyspnea
- Dysuria, edema
- Scant perspiration

Disorders in Circulating the Waterways
- Phlegm, mucus
- Edemas, especially in the face, eyelids, and upper region of body

Body Regions
- Skin and body hair
- Voice
- Nose, throat
- Nasal mucus

Disorders
- Skin: rough, dry; surface of the body is vulnerable to attacks from external pathogenic factors (Wind, Cold, Heat, Dampness, dryness, summer heat); open pores (increased perspiration)
- Body hair: withered, dry, dull
- Voice: weak, quiet, no desire to speak, dysphonia
- Nose: stuffed up, lost sense of smell, flaring nostrils, rhinorrhea
- Throat: pain, dryness, irritation, infections
- Breathing: respiratory difficulty, sneezing, snoring

Kidney Organ

Location	Lumbar area
Element with which it relates	Water
Hours	5 p.m. to 7 p.m.
Season	Winter
Time of day	Midnight
Associated Viscera	Bladder

Physiological Functions

Jing Storage

- Storage of innate Jing and surplus acquired Jing (Essence from food that was not used to cover the organism's needs)
- Maturation of sexual functions, fecundity, growth, and development
- Blood production (bone marrow, as an aspect of Jing), immunity (from Jing)

Govern Water and Fluids

- Transport of the pure portion that goes to nourishing tissues
- Transformation and excretion of the muddy portion
- Evaporation
- Fluids in the deep regions of the body
- The Lung regulates fluids in the body's peripheral regions; Spleen extracts liquids from food

Reception of Qi

- Allows for full, harmonious, and effective breathing

Dysfunctions

Disorders in Storing Jing

- Dysfunctions in growth and development (delayed growth in children, mental and/or physical malformations)
- Diminished sexual Energy, impotence, sterility
- Premature aging (tooth loss, premature graying)
- Disturbances in Blood production
- Reduced immunity
- Lack of vitality, weak legs

Disorders in Governing Water and Fluids

- Edemas
- Too little urination (oliguria) or too much (polyuria), frequent urination (pollakiuria)
- Urinary incontinence, terminal dripping
- Painful urination
- Failure of kidneys to produce urine (anuria)

Disorders in Receiving Energy
- Labored breathing (dyspnea)
- Asthma, breathlessness

Body Regions
- Marrow
- Brain
- Bones
- Teeth
- Ears
- Inferior orifices (anus, urethra, genital)
- Saliva

Disorders
- Bones: weak, fragile, difficulty mending broken bones
- Ears: deafness, ringing
- Teeth: dull, dry, stark, insistent cavities, weak, loose, falling out
- Brain: vertigo, insomnia, poor memory, inability to concentrate, reduced vision
- Marrow: Blood deficiency, malnourished bones and teeth
- Inferior orifices: disorders in defecation, urination, and reproduction; spermatorrhea
- Saliva: tendency to spit

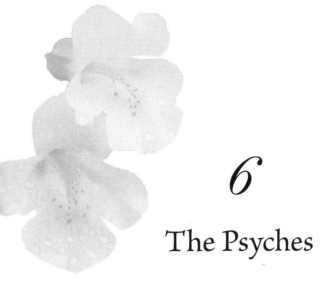

6

The Psyches

The Visceral Spirits, or *Wu Shen* (Five Spirits), keep residence in the Five Organs, each one of which provides them with a home, allowing them to carry out their functions.

They say that it is Shen (Spirit) expressing itself through these five forms.

Shen is the most subtle, most spiritual aspect of the human being; thanks to it, we are conscious of our existence. Its origin is celestial, which is why it is said that light, in the human being, is borrowed from the Heavens.

Dr. Bach tells us a bit more about it, in chapter 2 of *Heal Thyself*, when he makes the example of the Sun as the source, with its rays of light, and conscious beings as particles at the end of those rays. If a ray separates from the Sun, it ceases to exist.

Shen is also the consciousness that organizes and configures the human being, deciding to express itself in the human form. It allows us to behave in ways that enable our constant communication with, and adaptation to, our environment.

Our emotional, psychological, and spiritual functioning occur thanks to Shen. It relates closely with our affective and emotional lives, allowing us to feel an Emotion while being conscious of it.

Shen lends coherency to the personality and synthesizes the

activity of the four other Shen. Each one of the five represents a particular viewpoint, tied to Wood, Fire, Earth, Metal, and Water.

Shen integrates mental, sensory, and sensitive aspects, equipping us so that, when communicating with the outside world, we can adapt ourselves in the best way possible to each given circumstance.

Although each Organ is the residence of each Shen, the Organs do not manage the life of the psyche; they just provide the material base so that each Shen can express itself.

The Five Shen and the Five Organs maintain relationships that are mutually influential, in such a way that they may coordinate themselves for the balanced functioning of the psychic and the physical.

For the purposes of our work, we will call the Five Shen, Psyches. We will thereby say that each Organ is related with a particular Psyche, as is charted below. Below we see which Organ houses which Psyche and the name given to it by the Chinese.

> The Liver houses *Hun*.
> The Heart keeps *Shen*.
> The Spleen is related to *Yi*.
> The Lung corresponds with *Po*.
> The Kidney relates with *Zhi*.

As Eric Marié states, in his book, *Compendio de Medicina China*, each one of the Five Shen "is in charge of a particular aspect of the personality, of Emotions and of specific manners of behavior."

The notions the Chinese have about the Five Shen are of great richness and depth. This book will deal with those aspects tied to emotional, mental, and psychological realms. The more classical, ancient concepts will be approached in upcoming works about the Daoist view with relation to the Flowers.

For now, we'll consider the balanced manifestation of each Psyche as an expression of the Virtues it lends us—which is as much as to say that imbalances, due to excessive or insufficient expression, can be viewed as "defects."

Many variables come into play so that in each person one Psyche or another shows more strength or weakness, or expresses itself in a more balanced way. The characteristics we observe in our clients will be derived from this point of view.

Hun

Hun is related to Wood and the Liver.

It is Hun who gives us the power to push, the impulse to begin an action. Hun makes it possible for us to set things in motion. Later we'll see that it's a different Psyche that sustains this action with continuity.

But it's not about a blind impulsive force, because thanks to Hun, we are also able to "see beyond," as in, to establish a strategy. It's not in vain that the Liver is considered the general who decides the strategy.

Vision and the impetus for action provide tools that make the creation and elaboration of projects possible.

When in balance, Hun gives us direction for planning our lives, which, seen from a transcendental perspective, implies finding a way to carry out our own life's purpose.

The instinct for the conservation of the species, instinctive intelligence, and exercising astuteness are all rooted in this Psyche.

Astuteness can be a very useful skill to meet the ends mentioned above. These days, though, astuteness is overused; there is a tendency to take advantage as much as possible for one's own benefit, not caring about what that might mean for other people and the environment. It's a part of greed, of wanting more for oneself and less for others.

Hun is also related with desires and passions: urges arise from him. Hun gives power to the word.

Through the relations it maintains with Blood and the Liver, this Psyche gives us imagination, vision, and dreams. It has an important role in the act of creating.

Just as Wood and the Liver seek to express themselves outwardly, Hun has to do with extroversion, with the capacity we have as humans to relate with one another.

Traumas, unresolved problems from the past, dissatisfaction, and repressed desires all provoke imbalances in the areas related to this Psyche.

When This Psyche Lacks Strength

When Hun lacks strength, impulse is weakened, with repercussions appearing in diverse forms in the various areas of this Psyche.

A state of irritability, anxiety, or frustration could arise as a product of not having the necessary impulse for action.

Frequent sighs, as are observed in the presence of sadness, may indicate a deficiency in this Psyche.

The person may be overcome with fear and shyness when a diminished outward impulse manifests itself as retraction, as a form of retreating into himself. These symptoms could also be present when the Gallbladder is weak.

Enthusiasm dies down, and with it, projects and desires do too. When the expansive force provided by a balanced Hun is weakened, everything begins to get smaller and turn inward, seeming impoverished and less creative, losing the richness of the unconscious realm.

Imagination also becomes poor. One feels isolated.

It becomes very difficult then to elaborate plans for the future and to organize daily life.

Rigidity of thought and body ensue as softness and flexibility, typical of Wood and a properly functioning Liver, are lost.

According to various contemporary authors, mentioned by Eduardo Alexander in his thesis, there is a reduced capacity to steer oneself toward one's own destiny and to makes plans for unfolding one's life in accordance with the development of one's potential. This can lead to states of depression, to a feeling of having lost the meaning of life.

When This Psyche Is Expressed in Excess

An increased attitude of rejecting and feeling rejected notably disrupts relations with others.

Sleep is disturbed and restlessness, nightmares, and violent dreams may appear.

What was introversion in a deficient Hun now becomes an overflowing and luxuriant imagination. Expansion becomes exaggerated, and the person is excessively extroverted. Projects, besides being exaggerated, may seem incoherent, and the person may have a considerable lack of control in her impulses, which could start to become a pattern.

Everything pushes outward and wants to grow.

Shen

Shen is related to Fire and the Heart.

As we noted at the beginning of this chapter, it is through Shen that we are able to perceive our own existence. Shen is consciousness, and it is this Spirit that provides us with the desire to express ourselves through living, the desire to be alive.

It is Shen who coordinates the psyche and gives coherence to the personality.

Eduardo Alexander tells us in his thesis that Shen is "related to the Heart and Fire, and represents the power to name which means the act of giving an identity both to things in the world and also, especially, to oneself. The phase of Fire represents the dawn of self-awareness."

Also, thanks to Shen, we can understand things and facts directly without having to go through the whole learning process. Shen shares with the previous Psyche, Hun, the realm of dreams, to which Shen adds the ability to sleep in and of itself.

When Shen is in balance, one finds oneself with a clear mind, expressed in coherent discourse. Serenity is also a sign that Shen is in balance.

When This Psyche Lacks Strength

A sense of proportion—that of a just perception of things and situations—is lost, which is to say that one has a diminished capacity for adapting to life's circumstances.

When the desire to exist, to be alive in this world, shrinks, the person may enter into depressive states and tend toward shyness. For the same reason, the person may be more inclined to be constantly complaining of feeling ill at ease.

Coherency of the personality may be lost, discourse becomes unintelligible, the mind becomes cloudy, and, in extreme cases, one may enter into the realm of insanity.

When This Psyche Is Expressed in Excess

In excess, Shen is expressed as state of euphoria marking the loss of serenity. Mental clarity is also disturbed, giving way to confusion and resulting in marked incoherence and disconnection.

Yi

Yi is related to Earth and the Spleen.

This Psyche corresponds with the learning process. It is the most mental of the Five Shen, and our capacities for study and reflection depend upon it.

Yi allows us to store what we've learned in our memory and to recover it when necessary. Yi gives us the faculty for generating concepts and the ability to enunciate them—to communicate the thoughts we've elaborated.

Through Yi we are able to comprehend, though in a way that's different from the kind of comprehension given to us by Shen. With Yi, our understanding is derived from a process of study, reflection, and incorporation.

In a larger sense, it allows us to take in experiences as we live them.

When This Psyche Lacks Strength

Evidently, the learning process becomes complicated. In Dr. Bach's postulates, learning life's lessons is a very important point, which is why keeping the Spleen balanced and functioning is one of our tasks in our work with Flower Essences. We can keep the Spleen balanced by regulating the Emotions that alter the Organ and by promoting the balanced aspects of its Psyche.

With a weak Yi, memory is notably reduced, and instead, ideas become fixed and difficult to circulate. Conceiving of and managing concepts gets harder, while getting confused becomes easier.

Worry and obsession start showing up in heavy doses. Ideas begin having less mobility, tending to become fixed.

Larch-type states may appear as an inferiority complex, and the person's marked, excessive altruism will blatantly call our attention.

When This Psyche Is Expressed in Excess

The degree of obsession increases considerably. The mind becomes populated with fixed ideas, experiences that spin round and round in the mental plane, indicating an imperious need for White Chestnut.

Then, as if the mind didn't have enough activity, a formidable Honeysuckle state may appear as the person gets stuck in thoughts about past experiences.

Po

Po is related to Metal and the Lung.

Whereas in Hun there is a tendency toward expansion and extroversion, Po's Movement is the opposite: delimitation, introversion, and a tendency toward condensation.

Po is what gives density to our body.

Consistent with what we've said so far about Po, we can see that this Psyche is the most corporal, the one that lets us perceive the limits of our body, and thanks to him we can feel our own physical structures: bones, muscles, internal organs, joints. Po grants us the capacity to perceive the internal sensations of our body and indicates its orientation, and that of its segments, in physical space. Po gives us information about our posture, our balance, and everything else we need to feel while we move through space, so we can do it with balance and direction.

This is the Psyche responsible for the illusion of separation from all that exists, providing us with a sense of individuality and feeding egocentricity, thus permitting the experience of human life. Po incites us with the desire to live for ourselves alone.

Balancing this Psyche, and helping us to return little by little to a sense of unity, is good work for the Flowers. Part of the human condition is that, at some point, we may feel separateness in a powerful way, but then once again incorporate a sense of unity, taking with us the experience of human life.

Po also participates in the capacity to adapt to the changes that happen throughout our lives. It helps us to avoid danger, thanks to our ability to feel our bodies. Some authors maintain that it allows us to choose, without the participation of consciousness awareness, that which we need for maintaining the life of the body. When expressed in harmony, Po maintains our will to live.

When This Psyche Lacks Strength

When Po expresses itself with less force, dark ideas of death and suicide grow within us.

Brutal and important life changes impair this Psyche's capabilities, and in turn it becomes more difficult to adapt to those changes.

The will to live is lost, and the processes of death and destruction are activated.

Apathy and the urge to abandon everything arise along with a great sense of vulnerability, sadness, and suffering.

We may make choices inappropriate for sustaining the life of the body.

Exaggerated jealousy and a desire for revenge are two aspects to keep in mind when talking with our clients, as both of these indicate disturbances in this Psyche.

When This Psyche Is Expressed in Excess

Eric Marié in his book *Compendio de Medicina China* says "as seen in the previous Psyche, [Yi], a marked obsessive tendency appears [when Po is in excess] corresponding to fear of the future."

Zhi

Zhi is related to Water and the Kidney.

Zhi confers the capacity for realization. The strength of will. That which allows us to firmly sustain the goals and objectives of Shen.

Zhi gives us the tenacity needed to persist and to achieve our goals without getting sidetracked by obstacles. Strength of character, of determination, depend upon this Psyche.

It equips us with perseverance, thanks to which the mind can center itself on the goals it set and can pursue them without distraction.

Zhi participates in self-affirmation, giving us authority and determination.

It is the will to live in relation to a purpose.

When This Psyche Lacks Strength

Firmness of character is lost and we become indecisive and overly changeable.

We lack access to the strength and the tools necessary for confronting difficulties, so we remain subjugated to these difficulties and become easily discouraged as a consequence of lacking the necessary strength to pursue our goals with steadfastness.

Fear and dread begin to appear.

We're no longer able to keep ourselves aligned with the objectives we've set for ourselves.

Angst and anxiety are frequent . . . the will to live dwindles . . . total apathy may ensue . . . the meaning of life is lost.

When This Psyche Is Expressed in Excess

Willpower, the strength to realize, turns into authoritarianism.

There is a tendency toward tyranny.

That which was tenacity becomes obstinacy.

Behavior is dreadful.

Suggestions for Working with the Psyches

We might note that the contents of the Psyches, such as they are described in this book, turn out to be familiar to Flower Essence Therapists. The capacities to realize, to evaluate, and to persist; learning difficulties; and the suffering that these areas create are what we find ourselves facing in our practice.

Let's take a look at some ways to make use of what we now know about the Psyches.

- Aspects of a balanced Psyche can serve as a guide to help us develop these qualities in the person consulting us by providing him or her with the related Flowers.
- We may recognize which Psyche is upset and work on balancing it.
- Once we have detected the Psyche or Psyches (not usually more than two) that have been out of balance since early childhood, we'll be able to see how the theme of this Psyche has repeated itself over the course of our client's lifetime. This is a very good way to work at the base of disorders and is probably related to the Virtue or Virtues that our client needs to be developing.

- Eduardo Alexander mentions, in his thesis, Lonny Jarret's* ideas regarding one's constitution as a sort of fixation that, stemming out of events happening early in life, keep one stuck in a singular interpretation of the world and of life. As such, Emotions accumulate, intoxicating the person. The way to work with one's constitution is through the Virtues. These allow us to reorganize the disturbed Emotions and to return to a more fluid mode of interpreting the world. No doubt the Flowers are a privileged tool for helping us to develop these Virtues. We can appreciate the relationship between these concepts, taken by Jarret from Daoism, and Dr. Bach's postulates. So, we need to detect from which Psyche the individual interprets the world and work with the individual to balance it and its corresponding Virtues. Just as in Bach's work, by developing the Virtue related to the lesson we are experiencing, everything else falls into place. The Virtues cannot be developed by force of will; instead, it is better to create an environment in which they may spring forth. In this sense, the Flowers are more than indicated, considering that they naturally, without our imposition, bring about a flourishing of the Virtues. Imposing the will usually has the opposite effect.
- If we accept that rigidity in the way a person exists in the world generates, among other things, emotional disturbances that crystallize as symptoms in the body, then, once we know which Psyche is needing work and relate it to its corresponding Organ, we have at our disposal all the relationships the Psyche and Organ maintain with the rest of the body. As such, we can investigate physical disorders with the added benefit of understanding how an imbalance in a determined Psyche generates pathologies. By giving the corresponding Flowers, our intent is to balance the Psyche, develop the Virtues, and, via this route, heal physical disorders.
- Working with the Psyches may also lead us to detect, in Bach's terms, the personality type of the person consulting us. The Twelve Healers can help us to balance the personality, though evidently we need to allow ourselves the freedom to work with all of the Flowers.

---

*[Jarret is the author of *Nourishing Destiny: The Inner Tradition of Chinese Medicine* (Stockbridge, Mass.: Spirit Path Press, 1999) and *The Clinical Practice of Chinese Medicine* (Stockbridge, Mass.: Spirit Path Press, 2006). —*Trans.*]

- If we look at the Lung's Psyche, we see that one of its themes is the ability to adapt to life's changes. We know that essences like Walnut, Star-of-Bethlehem, Rock Water, and other Flowers related to rigidity can be helpful. But we also get an idea of how difficulties in adapting to life's changes can influence areas corresponding with the Lung, which may affect body fluids, skin, and the large intestine just as much as breathing. So we see how, in this case, the essences mentioned above may indirectly improve the Lung's functioning.
- Continuing with the example of the Lung's Psyche, its related Virtue is rectitude, having to do with a balance between that which I take and that which I lose, among other aspects. Certain Flowers become evident like Vine, Chicory, Centaury, Clematis, and Heather.

In table 6.1, the Organs are given with their corresponding Psyches and Virtues.

TABLE 6.1. CORRESPONDENCES AMONG THE ORGANS

Organ	Psyche	Virtues
Liver	Hun	Benevolence, Kindness, Goodness
Heart	Shen	Courtesy, Correctness, Propriety
Spleen	Yi	Trustworthiness, Confidence, Faith, Integrity, Honesty, Honor
Lung	Po	Rectitude, Justice
Kidney	Zhi	Wisdom, Intelligence

Part 2

Bach Flowers from a Chinese Medical Perspective

The following texts about the Bach Remedies were written within the framework of the seminar "Las Flores de Bach: Cuatro Miradas Integradoras" (Bach Flower Remedies: Four Integrative Viewpoints).

In this series of smaller seminars, we cover the Twelve Healers, the Seven Helpers, the Ten Trees, and the last Nine Flowers. This series has been offered without interruption from 2006 to date.

Organized by Dr. Ricardo Orozco's Institut Anthemon in Barcelona, the seminar is given by the professors Ricardo Orozco, Jordi Cañellas, Josep Guarch, and myself. We take a look at the Flowers from the viewpoints of contemporary psychology and emotional intelligence, the Transpersonal Patterns, the signature of the Flowers, astrology, and Chinese Medicine.

The reader will find, throughout these texts, references to these dear friends to whom I am profoundly grateful for the work shared.

I have taken for granted that the reader already has an understanding of the Bach Remedies, but if this is not the case, there are numerous books available to help acquire basic or in-depth knowledge.

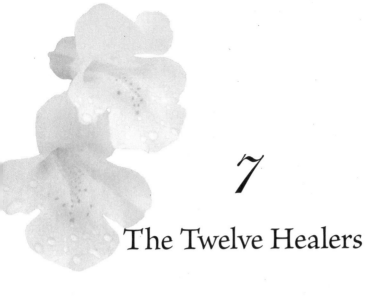

7

The Twelve Healers

Impatiens

Organs, Emotions, Psyche

Although the form through which each Flower type expresses itself in the world influences the totality of the person, it is still possible to observe tendencies affecting certain Organs and areas. Knowledge of these tendencies allows us to ask questions to deepen our perception, consider aspects that sometimes even the person consulting us is unable to distinguish, and prevent possible disorders.

In the Impatiens type, the Liver, Heart, and Kidney, among other Organs, may be affected.

The Liver

The characteristic impatience, irritability, indignation, anxiety, and restlessness of the Impatiens personality all fully impact this Organ. These attitudes and Emotions likewise foment the stagnation of Liver Energy and the accumulation of Heat.

Acceleration is a characteristic effect of Heat, and likewise, Heat generates acceleration, establishing a self-perpetuating cycle. It is this pathogenic factor that creates a base for the fits of rage that, as Ricardo comments, may be quick to rise and just as quick to disappear, revealing aspects of Wind.

Wind manifests itself in Impatiens personalities as fits of rage, tics, nervous finger movements, and other possible symptoms. We'll look at these aspects of Wind in detail further ahead.

The tension and nervousness we see in the Impatiens type arise out of the way the personality experiences obstacles, felt to be put there by the slowness of others. Just as Jordi comments, Impatiens moves by the Energy of impulse. This Energy, in nature, is provided by Wood, and in the body, by the Liver.

This is to say that in Impatiens's case, much is being asked of the Liver; it is being challenged to sustain an impulse disproportionate to its balanced functioning and to deal with the stagnation provoked by frustration and other Liver-related Emotions. Like the expansiveness of Wood, one of the Liver's functions is the free expression of oneself. The intensity of the Emotions at play increases when unable to freely express.

This Organ's Psyche participates in an important way, given that it, too, provides the impulse for action and the driving force of urges. When out of balance, it favors rigidity and difficulty in relating with others, creating rejection—the person is both extroverted and self-centered. Impulsiveness is less controllable and can lead to compulsion.

The tension, cramps, and stiff muscles that we see in Impatiens-type persons find part of their origin in the difficulty the Liver has in distributing Blood to the parts of the body that need it due to activity, leaving these parts poorly supplied, thus provoking the described symptoms.

The Heart

Anxiety, lack of serenity, acceleration, nervousness, and tension—all typical of the Impatiens type—can affect the Heart.

Heat influences Blood (which is the material base for Spirit and the mind), and opens the door to symptoms that can range from simple anxiety and restlessness to severe mental disorders. Mental acceleration increases Fire, which, as Dr. Bach mentioned, could lead the Impatiens person be cruel.

Impatiens Flower Essence provides serenity and regulates Heat (among other aspects) thus favoring the balanced expression of the Heart's Psyche, smoothing out the path for: becoming conscious of oneself, becoming conscious of one's internal nature, and getting in contact with one's path in life.

The Kidney

Anxiety and acceleration disturb the Kidney. It is this Organ that, generally speaking, controls Fire, given that it corresponds with the Water element and manages the root of Water and Fire within the organism. When in balance, the Kidney prevents Heat from accumulating in the Liver: this Heat, if not regulated, will end up being transmitted to the Heart. Proper activity of the Kidney will prevent Heat from shooting up to the body's upper parts and dilapidating body fluids and Energy.

Virtues

Benevolence is the Virtue related to the Liver's Psyche. Balanced functioning of the Liver favors the cultivation of this Virtue, which implies the capacity to make room for others in one's life while at the same time allowing them to develop their own life's plan. In his book, *Flores de Bach: 38 descripciones dinámicas* (Bach Flower Remedies: 38 Dynamic Descriptions), Ricardo explains the meaning of the lesson to be learned by the Impatiens type, *forgiveness,* noting that it is sometimes translated to Spanish as *indulgence,* and how that relates to self-awareness. This lesson is highly relevant for developing Benevolence as a Virtue, and is also related to the Heart's Psyche, which provides the capacity for self-awareness.

Jordi tells us that Impatiens is an invasive plant that moves other species out of its way, which is the opposite attitude that the Virtue promotes.

The Liver's Psyche, when in balance, regulates this tendency.

Disorders That May Be Present

- Digestive disturbances, such as belching, vomiting, diarrhea, poor assimilation, abdominal distension, colic
- Pain in various parts of the body, in some cases piercing; pain that radiates and erratic pains
- Inflammation; chest, abdomen, and groin complaints
- Vertigo
- Tics, convulsions, cramps

- Stiff muscles, headaches
- Vision and hearing problems; ringing in the ears
- Sleep trouble
- Menstrual complaints; pain and swelling of the breasts
- Accelerated breathing and heartbeat

Comments

The fact that Impatiens Flower Essence is helpful in treating Heat helps us to understand its action on inflammation and anxiety. The essence also favors the balanced expression of the Heart's and Liver's Psyches. It probably also steers Energy toward the lower parts of the body.

Scleranthus is among the essences that can help Impatiens, regulating the time gap between Impatiens personalities and other people. Holly and Vervain, together with Water Violet and Rock Water, collaborate to modulate Heat. Cherry Plum can help dissolve stagnancy.

Two practices that could favor the path for spiritual growth and could have a very healing influence on Impatiens personalities are:

- cultivating a circular perception of time to mitigate the excessive linear experience of it
- doing or making something without looking toward any concrete result, and doing it just *because,* with no purpose in mind

Mimulus

Organs, Emotions, Psyche

This Flower has extensive influence on the Organs and their territories, due possibly to the fact that the type of fixation and Emotions that it treats are related to very primary areas of the human being, such as fear and its related territory.

Let's look at which Organs may be touched by Mimulus's way of being in the world.

The Liver

Liver disturbances may be common given that many of the Mimulus person's Emotions and ways of being damage the capacity to softly and uniformly move Energy and fluids, a function that assists the development of multiple processes in the human being.

The Transpersonal Pattern is very clear here, synthesized at many levels in the Mimulus person as a retraction of impulse. This intent to slow or detain the river of Energy has consequences that are expressed in different areas depending on the person's constitution and history.

Introversion and shyness, fear, frustration, depressive states, and mistrust also harm this Organ. As Ricardo mentions, bitterness and resentment are Mimulus's way of compensating for these states. Anxiety likewise creates imbalances in this and other Organs.

When—as a consequence of the above-mentioned sentiments and modes—Energy, Blood, and fluids do not circulate smoothly, rigidity of body and mind sets in. The characteristic softness of the Liver is lost. Fluids, and denser substances like mucus and cysts, may accumulate in various parts of the body.

Persistent stagnation of Energy creates Heat, gestating an irritability that can evolve into resentment.

The Liver's Psyche provides, among other aspects, the capacity for extroversion and the impulse for initiating action. If these qualities lack sufficient strength to be put into play, the Emotion that naturally arises is frustration; this is a clear consequence of the inability to express one's plans, feelings and opinions.

The Spleen

The Mimulus-type person spends a great deal of time worrying and thinking. He attempts to prevent and control circumstances by anticipating them in thought. In the best possible case, these thoughts are a means of using logic against fear by opposing fear with reason.

The problem is that the Energy used for these processes comes from the Spleen, in detriment to food distribution and assimilation, and likewise to the production and distribution of Blood and Energy.

Debility in the Spleen's Psyche prepares the ground for a growth in shyness and sense of inferiority.

A large portion of Mimulus's Energy is lost in the need to keep everything under as much control as possible.

The Lung

The pessimistic, negative contents of Mimulus's thoughts and worries impact this Organ. The same occurs with melancholy and depressive states. Excess introversion may originate as much in a deficient Liver Psyche as in disorders of the Lung's Psyche. When there is a deficiency in the latter, the ability to adapt to life's changes is lost, a tendency toward isolation grows, and the person is more vulnerable.

The Kidney

The relationship between fear and the Kidneys is quite well-known; many people have observed that one of the effects of fear can be urinary incontinence.

Fear causes Energy to descend. The legs and knees feel weak and shaky. The Kidney's Energy loses solidity and shrinks. There may be fecal incontinence given that the Kidney controls the inferior orifices: anus and urethra.

We could say that fear has many effects; it ages, takes away strength and immunity, deteriorates bones, delays the knitting of fractures, weakens the lumbar area, and, when it is extreme, creates paralysis (Rock Rose).

If persistent, fear can upset one's growth rate, sexual vigor and reproductive capacity, and can also create Blood deficiency disorders and imbalances in quantity and frequency of urination.

When edemas are present, we might consider fear as a factor. Shallow breathing may lead us in the same direction, as may asthma and respiratory fatigue.

Weakness in the Kidney's Psyche will be found in areas related to authority, affirmation, and determination. This Psyche must be strengthened in order to gain security and reduce vulnerability.

Kidney imbalances can be observed when fear-related Emotions arise, such as apprehension, phobia, cowardice.

In some cases, to compensate for retraction, audacity may appear. But boldness is difficult to sustain as it uses up the little Energy that this personality type has in the first place. In other cases, as Ricardo mentions, a Vine attitude appears and may persist over time provided the person in question is not a Mimulus type with a weak Kidney constitution, evident in the person's fragile appearance (curved posture and paleness). This Organ is in charge of giving strength and solidity to the physical body. Just as Josep Guarch states with respect to Capricorn, bones are supported by Kidney Energy.

The Lung, Spleen, and Kidney have a clear participation in the Waterways, which is to say, in the circulation and distribution of organic fluids. Mimulus, as a state, can arise from disturbances in various Organs and Viscera. A deficient Gallbladder predisposes a person to fearfulness, shyness, vulnerability, and gullibility. In cases of Liver, Heart, or Kidney weakness, and with Blood deficiencies, the person is predisposed to feel fear.

Virtues

Wisdom is the Virtue corresponding to the Kidney. It provides balance between excessive caution and daredevilry. This Organ also gives us the capacity to keep calm when posed with the fear that arises when facing the unknown. The Spleen bestows us with the capacity to maintain our integrity while at the same time paying attention to the exchange and distribution of vital Energy shared with another person, guaranteeing the integrity of both parties.

Comments

Heather Essence can help the Mimulus person not be so self-centered in his worries. Other essences can help provide Energy, like Centaury, Clematis and Olive, as well as those that help with stagnation, like Crab Apple, Willow, Chicory, and Cherry Plum.

I agree with Josep when he says that Mimulus rejects himself, believing that others are going to evaluate him using the same measure; that is why he acts, as Ricardo describes, "with a clear Avoidant conduct meant to protect him from ridicule, humiliation, and above all, negative judgment and rejection."

That which is unfathomable, dangerous, and mysterious finds its home in Water, and the Mimulus plant, as we see in its signature, lives at the edge of running water. The Mimulus person is often surprised to find that he has the strength and resources for facing that which he fears. At those times, like the plant, he deepens his roots so he won't be carried away in the current. The problem is that he often discovers his capacities in the midst of full-blown catastrophe and doesn't keep this awareness of his strength during times of peace.

Clematis

Organs, Emotions, Psyche

The Kidney

The will to live while keeping a perception of the meaning of life are aspects of the Kidney's Psyche. If the Kidney's Psyche lacks strength, the root of willpower is affected, the meaning of life is lost, there's a sense of discouragement, and it becomes easy to fall into extreme apathy. The mind is unable to apply itself toward goals.

The Spleen

The disruption suffered by the Spleen shows up as: poor memory, scarce intake of life experiences, weak capacity for attention and concentration, muscular weakness, and other disorders.

Nutrients derived from the earth reach us through this Organ, which increases our material being and thus implies a sort of grounding. The Spleen also helps produce Blood that, as we will see below, influences the capacity to be grounded.

The Lung

When disturbed, the Lung manifests (through its Psyche) a weak survival instinct and little will to live. The reflex to protect oneself from danger is diminished. The person demonstrates poor adaptation to change and desires distance, wishing to abandon everything, and showing disinterest and vulnerability that may manifest in the body as reduced immunity.

Our ability to perceive our senses—to experience sensations, thus permitting contact with the outside world and with others—resides in the Lung. Sight and hearing depend upon this aspect of the Lung (and also on the Liver and Kidney, respectively). The Lung's Psyche is related to being fully in the body in order to perceive and to take action in the world. The Spirit of the Lung, *Po,* is the Psyche in charge of forming the body, and Metal, the element corresponding to the Lung, provides the Energy for materialization. Jordi assigns to Clematis the "Cosmic Principle of Manifestation."

This Organ manages a type of Energy that is formed by:

- The Energy the Lung obtains from the air
- The Energy coming from the subtle Essence of food, having been elaborated by the Spleen.

This is to say that it orchestrates the union of celestial and earthly Energies into one single Energy. This unified Energy is one of the Energies that circulates throughout the channels, nourishing the whole organism.

Clematis-type persons have a tendency toward some degree of paleness, indicating a deficiency of Energy, Blood, or both.

The Lung's activity also permits grounding through its relationship with the Kidney toward whom Energy and fluids descend.

The Liver

The Liver holds the potential for balancing the Clematis person's "flight," transforming a soaring imagination into creative action, nourished by the riches of the unconscious. Here, dreaming serves realization—to dream in order to create something practical.

Blood holds vital importance in grounding a person. It is said that Blood is the vehicle of the Spirit, the material base for the mind. When there is a Blood deficiency, particularly in the Liver, the mind wanders, one daydreams, the meaning of life unravels, and the person no longer pays attention to goals. When the light of consciousness and presence of mind are not in the here and now, the body becomes uninhabited.

The Liver's Psyche provides us with the capacity to find our true path in order to travel through life in accordance with our destiny.

Virtues

Benevolence is the Virtue that corresponds to Clematis Flower Essence. Cultivating benevolence benefits the Liver, permitting the realization of the lesson that the Clematis person came into this life to learn.

Comments

When one lacks Energy, many vital processes fade, and the disorders this produces, when long-standing, become intertwined and feed off each other. A sense of being grounded deteriorates, and the tendency to "space out" increases. This gives way to symptoms that are frequently present in Clematis-type persons like weariness, apathy, and diminished strength in the arms and legs. The face is pale. Immunity also fades, and the person has more difficulty adapting to changes in the weather. This reduced capacity for adaptation is understandable given that the Clematis person takes very poor note of what's happening in the present, complicating the adaptive process. It is a very marked state of abandonment of the body that doesn't quite reach total abandonment (though the Clematis person wouldn't be worried if it were). The production of Blood and body fluids is disrupted, as is circulation.

Clematis Flower Essence tones Energy, favoring circulation of both Blood and Energy, and it's in this sense, as Ricardo notes, that it works on cold feet.

It's probably helpful for the Clematis person to connect with a meaning in life, to discover her own purpose in the world. Wild Oat could be handy in orientation. Maybe this way, as Josep comments, the person can connect with some of the possibilities available for developing her innate potential.

Agrimony

Organs, Emotions, Psyche

Joy has a marvelous effect on the person as a whole. It brings relaxation and calms the mind. It improves prospects for being nourished and increases immunity. Blood and Energy circulate better, so communication between the various parts of the body and the mind are optimal. Joy, in short, fully sets us in harmony.

We are talking about a spontaneous and authentic kind of joy, not the kind that rises up against hell and high water, hiding beneath its surface less benign and more painful Emotions or simply those Emotions whose carrier classifies, even unconsciously, as unpresentable.

This is where things become complicated for Agrimony.

The Heart

The constant excitement and euphoria, a schedule filled with activities, and the excess consumption of food, alcohol, and drugs that the Agrimony type entertains generate internal Heat, which, over time, can give way to deficiency and debility. This lifestyle is injurious to the Heart, who, as *Emperor* of the Organs (Heart, Spleen, Lung, Kidney, Liver) and Viscera (Small Intestine, Stomach, Large Intestine, Bladder, Gallbladder), may, when imbalanced, reign harshly over its subjects. This explains in part why an Agrimony state is the origin of numerous disorders and severely degenerative chronic illnesses.

Anxiety also engenders Heat and is at the same time engendered by it. Once again the Heart may be paying the consequences, though anxiety may equally affect the Spleen, Lung, and Kidney.

The Heart's Psyche provides, among other things, coherency to the personality, consciousness, and a perception of one's own existence. It coordinates the whole of the human psyche. When in balance, the state that emerges is one of serenity and mental clarity; when not, these qualities are interrupted by euphoria and incoherency.

Such is the impetus that the Agrimony person has to distance herself from herself that, rather than allowing the Heart to reign in her impulses, she lets herself get carried away with excesses.

The Agrimony person suffers from a serious dissociation which eliminates from her consciousness many of the contents of her person, reducing coherency and integration of the personality, leading to unease, restlessness, inability to discern, and a want for peace.

The person seeks to find peace through negating conflict and fatiguing the Emotions associated with the Heart, exercising joy at all hours until it becomes a mask, a defect.

Harmony, a natural fruit of authentic joy, slips clean past joy-by-decree.

The Spleen

The Heart is not the only Organ affected given that Agrimony's way of being generates a cumulus of Emotions that impact other Organs which, when they become imbalanced, sustain their respective negative Emotions.

Worry, by draining the Spleen, weakens digestion and assimilation (already strained by Agrimony's dietary habits), bringing weariness (it gets little rest) and an accumulation of mucus and substances that can lead to, for example, Gallbladder or Kidney stones, or respiratory and Heart disorders.

The Spleen's Energy becomes blocked, making learning in every sense of the word more difficult, while also increasing obsession.

The Kidney

Fear affects the root of the human being—the Kidney and its entire sphere of action. And there, in the impenetrable, hidden place of Water (the Kidney belongs to this element), that which is most essentially nourishing is found, guarded. In the depths of Water—in the darkness of that which is undifferentiated—primary vitality and human potential are hidden. And here we have revealed Agrimony's imbalance between Fire and Water, Heart and Kidney. The red and black of the plant's rhizome expresses the same: consciousness and that which is seen under the light of day versus that which is hidden in the depth of night, in the darkness of the Kidney. This is one of Agrimony's most important dilemmas.

Joy and, hidden beneath it, fear—the unpleasant, the unknown—reveal this disconnected relationship between the Kidney and the Heart. That which is hidden nourishes and gives life to that which is manifest. Water is the root that prevents Fire from escaping upward and debilitating the person.

When no room is made for darkness, very valuable parts of oneself are killed along with it. The imbalance it generates ends up growing into an even bigger darkness that, furthermore, doesn't cease to exist just because it isn't being seen.

Virtues

As in the case of joy, the Virtues corresponding to the Heart are exercised in a forced march; thus courtesy and correction become worn out. Virtue, when exaggerated, gives birth to defect.

The Agrimony type needs to connect with authentic internal peace. And it will not be achieved by maintaining a lack of communication between the Heart and Kidney.

In the Kidney—in the very substance of the body, in the depth of the unconscious—we find the buried treasure that is the unique potential conferred to the person and the path to follow for developing it.

The bad news for the Agrimony person is that, in order to activate this potential, he must do exactly what he does not want to do. He must bring the consciousness of the Heart down into the depths, given that this interaction between the Heart's capacity for becoming conscious and the potential found in the Kidney is the way toward self-knowledge and toward putting into play the potential that awaits activation, driven by consciousness.

The Heart's and Kidney's Virtues must be used to direct one's will toward self-knowledge. Expressed in the Daoist tradition, the above process is known as "driving Fire down into Water," bringing consciousness toward the unimaginable in order to activate one's potential.

Comments

It is quite possible that the Agrimony person generate Heat, appearing as skin conditions, hemorrhages, insomnia, restlessness, accelerated metabolism, carbuncles, canker sores (quite torturous*), urinary disorders, fevers, and fever convulsions. The list is long, and we can investigate these disorders in the Agrimony person. The Flower Essence is useful for treating this Heat.

Another body region to keep in mind is the intestines. Both the Large and Small Intestines may be affected by Agrimony's lifestyle.

An application that may be of interest to us, inscribed within the essence's action as a catalyst, is to use it in processes that manifest themselves as normal and healthy on the outside but hide serious disorders deeper on the inside. For example, wounds that appear healthy on the surface but underneath contain pus, hidden hemorrhages, hidden septic points.

Also, taking the essence in processes in which the root of the complaint is unclear—processes that present contradictory symptoms that are difficult to bring together into a coherent story—allows us to dismiss appearances and define the origin.

Chicory

Organs, Emotions, Psyche

Let's take the "sticky" aspect inherent in Chicory. This is a factor that detains, slows, and somehow dirties the emotional sphere.

The latex found in the root is an unseen part of the plant. Likewise, people who fall within this profile do not see themselves as clingy but

---

*[*Torture* is the Transpersonal Pattern developed by Ricardo Orozco, also mentioned by Dr. Bach. —*Trans.*]

rather as wellsprings that let love flow left and right. If clinging fails to retain the other person, they become coarse, like the plant's stem. The data from the plant's signature are truly illuminating.

The Liver

The Chicory person's conduct, based on the need to control his environment, for reasons that my colleagues have explained very well,* seriously obstructs the free flow of Energy, Blood, and fluids. This endangers the Liver, which, as we've seen, suffers the consequences of each Flower type's lack of flexibility and fluidity.

Dr. Bach himself tells us about this obstruction in relation to greed. He states, "Exactly as we thwart another life, be it old or young, so must that re-act upon ourselves. If we limit their activities, we may find our bodies limited with stiffness" (Howard and Ramsell, *Original Writings of Edward Bach*, 56). Due to their great neediness, Chicory types try to "rule the world" (that of their affective environment and its surrounding townships), interfering with the development of others' lives, exerting effort to twist the paths of others for their own benefit. Something which we all know doesn't come for free.

Emotions like frustration and contained aggression influence the Organ in question, contributing to more stagnation. The result: fluid retention, edemas, and Blood stagnation, as may be observed in varicose veins and menstrual complications.

Emotions that are retained and stored for a long time can become Fire, so any irritability may quickly turn into anger, which becomes progressively more explosive. The Chicory person's need to dissimulate her hostility increases internal pressure, possibly turning into a full-blown Cherry Plum state.

This tension settles in the jaws, the throat, the chest, the rib cage and sides (remember the rigid structure of the plant's stem), the groin, and the breasts. It can also generate involuntary movements in different parts of the body.

It is not unusual for the Chicory person to suffer from insomnia. Anxiety increases, as does nervousness and further dissatisfaction.

---

*[Jordi Cañellas, for example, says the Chicory person feels empty inside, as expressed in the plant's hollow stem, which relates to the self, the ego. —*Trans.*]

Depression due to stagnation is presented and may increase with Heat.

Creating here a short and not at all exhaustive list of Emotions and attitudes that tend to be present in Chicory types and that affect the Liver, we find: anger, jealousy, explosiveness, tension, hate, vindictiveness, envy, irritability, frustration, rigidity, invasion. What is more, this Organ is in charge of maintaining emotional stability. So we get an idea of the work overload to which the Liver is subjected.

This Organ's Psyche oscillates between extremes, giving rise to its defects. When it becomes weak, sadness appears, along with a feeling of isolation and turning inward, sighs, depression, and fear.

If pushed to the limit, interpersonal relationships will tend to become complicated with harsh remarks, rejection, and feeling rejected.

The Liver carries a certain weight in gynecological problems.

The Gallbladder may also be disturbed, generating part of the vulnerability that the Chicory person feels with respect to his or her loved ones.

The Spleen

Another way to clog up Energy circulation is through self-centered obsession.

The systematic self-referencing present in the Chicory type keeps Energy in a loop, making stickiness and clinginess more powerful. This makes it very difficult to learn the lesson at hand, given that negative aspects tend to stick around and regenerate themselves over and over, passing from the body to the Emotions to the mind and back again. The tendency is toward chronic problems that are difficult to eliminate.

The "stickiness" appears as leucorrhea, mucus, or nodules in the breasts. Digestion is also disturbed with an erratic appetite; there may be belching, nausea, and epigastric upset.

Resentment in particular supports the accumulation of substances, creating imbalance in the Liver's and Spleen's functions.

Exaggerated caretaking and nutrition, increased worry, overprotection, and invasion in the life of the other person all harm the Spleen. It could go as far as a ruminant state, with a great tendency to exaggerate, which is cousin to susceptibility.

Lung

is another Organ that may be disturbed in Chicory persons.

Jealousy, desire for revenge, sadness, and vulnerability appear when the Lung's Psyche is weak.

But it is also this Psyche who allows us to exercise the Virtue that helps us maintain a balance between what we gain and what we lose, what we accumulate and what we eliminate.

It has an influence in the value we place upon relationships in our lives. Both the Lung and the Large Intestine have an influence on our capacity to let go—to release without losing what is valuable, what nourishes.

Virtues

Once again, benevolence is the Virtue to cultivate; remember that it is the Virtue that lets us include others in our life, but without restricting the development of their own particular path, their own life's plan.

Also, faith and confidence, as well as integrity and reciprocity, which favor the exchange of vital force between one another, guaranteeing the integrity of both parties.

On occasion, the Chicory person uses these Virtues as a mask to come in contact with other people, thus dissimulating the Emotions and intentions that are truly driving him or her.

Comments

Ear, eye, and skin problems (many times with suppurations) and a bitter flavor in the mouth may be some of the imbalances in Chicory.

It is a very useful essence for treating Liver Energy stagnation, Heart imbalances, Dampness disorders: nodules, cholesterol, mucus (anywhere it is found in the body), and white and sticky vaginal discharge. It helps Crab Apple with thick, sticky suppurations in any part of the body.

Agrimony Essence may foment a perception of what the Chicory person does not see in herself, which she buries deep in her unconscious mind. In balanced situations, Wood's Energy flows into Fire where its maximum expansive action should take place—an opportunity for love to reach every corner and every angle without restrictions. If stagnation is serious, this Movement does not take place, and what happens instead is an increase in Fire, not the love kind but the kind that burns, accelerates, and irritates. When fluids cannot flow, they become thick and accumulate. Taking Chicory Flower Essence, averting stagnation, gives water back its free-flowing potential.

Vervain

Organs, Emotions, Psyche

The Liver

Like Wood, the Liver seeks to extend itself it every direction with nothing holding it back. If Metal and the Lung's activity do not put the brakes on the Liver, it unfolds indomitably. This is exaggeration.

When the Liver is out of balance, the person acts without any thought mediation, letting himself be carried away by the expansive Energy that pushes, so what ought to be impulse for action turns into a sort of gale. This impulsiveness is commanded by rigid thought with a transgressor Spirit, giving rise to difficulties with boundaries—*what may be done and what may not be done.* Impulse is more difficult to control. Projects are exaggerated; there is no slowing down imagination and thoughts. Heat increases, and with it, tension and a tendency toward irritability, extremism, and hyperactivity. This very situation multiplies the propensity for indignation. Intolerance is much higher and may be expressed as a front to those who do not share the Vervain person's latest headline ideas.

The Heat and tension that are produced in the Liver may generate auditory disorders (the Vervain type does not listen because he is preaching), otitis, strong headaches; Energy ascends and, along with it, Blood, increasing the risk of a cerebrovascular accident. The face may be red, strained; there may be hemorrhages like nosebleed and possible insomnia and hypertension.

It is very difficult for the Vervain person to exercise diplomacy, and all this fullness of expression prevents him from utilizing the Liver's capacity to develop strategies.

The flexibility that this Organ bestows turns into rigidity, both physical and mental.

The Blood held in the Liver cannot be sent to the parts of the body that require it for implementing harmonious, coordinated Movements.

In healthy conditions, the Liver supports the lesson that corresponds to Vervain, predisposing him to feel spontaneously tolerant.

The Heart

Such powerful expansion of Energy from the Liver, creating abundant fuel for Fire, ascends and disseminates in all directions, bringing us to the Heart's territory. But it is a region devastated by Fire, without any vestige of balance.

A moderate level of excess could be seen as excitability, a constant want for stimuli, and strong Emotions. As Ricardo states, Vervain types seek danger, for example in extreme sports, and seek it in ever more powerful and exciting forms.

The Vervain person becomes unyielding to the point of rebellion and possibly hard enough to be cruel. Decidedly maniacal.

Ricardo comments that Vervain types can go so far as to sacrifice their lives, a maximum exaggeration of the capacity to handle extremes and cruelty, turned against themselves. An extreme way to destroy the ego.

Heat, on the other hand, stimulates and accelerates thought and speech—the impetus in the transmission of ideas. But moral consciousness is diminished.

Energy must be brought down, and the bitter flavor can accomplish this while also removing Heat. Water Violet Essence turns out to be very useful, supporting Vervain Essence's action in reducing Heat.

Virtues

Vervain imbalances manifest themselves as an exaggeration of Wood and Fire Energy. So attitudes are imposed on others who feel violated and invaded—when not directly dragged—by the virulence that the Vervain type displays. The Vervain person needs to connect with Wood and Fire Energy through their corresponding Virtues: benevolence, corresponding to the Liver (as we've mentioned in relation to other essences), to give space to others without annulling them, without taking them as if they were objects for manipulating; propriety, corresponding to the Heart, to perceive the adequacy of his actions within the social context in which he is immersed and in relation to his own life's plan.

Comments

It is said that it is important to review what one considers to be one's Virtues. All sorts of injustices have been committed in Virtues' name.

Cerato

Organs, Emotions, Psyche

Cerato-type people find themselves lost. They are disconnected from the part of themselves that holds their essential being, the part that allows them to connect with (in Bach's terms) their soul. They have no other option than to seek outside themselves. Such little value does the Cerato person give to what comes from inside that she needs social conventions to laboriously construct an artificial self that, what is more, changes all too frequently.

The Kidney

Lacking the strength that the Kidney and its Psyche can provide, the Cerato person is very flighty, possibly even docile enough to be easily influenced.

But, by empowering Kidney Energy, her indecisive and changeable character gives way to affirmation and her own authority. It will no longer be so easy to win her over with external authority because she now recognizes her own internal authority. The mind, much more centered, supports the completion of set goals. Determination increases. The fear that arises facing disorientation begins to diminish.

A balanced Kidney Psyche provides firmness and a reference point, allowing one to make comparisons and decisions based on one's own parameters.

Gallbladder

The Gallbladder helps us to modulate the influence that our environment has on us, strengthening determination and the capacity for making judgments, and thus, the capacity for making decisions. The services that a strong Gallbladder performs for a Cerato type are the following: diminishing a propensity for hypochondria and somatization, diminishing gullability, mitigating doubt, helping to act in consequence with decisions made. Some disorders of this Viscera can be approached using this Flower Essence.

The Spleen

Lack of confidence is also present, and whatever form it takes, it affects the Spleen's performance. Digestive processes are upset, Blood disorders may appear, lack of Energy, muscle weakness, and other related imbalances.

On the learning and intellectual plane, disturbances appear related to memory, concentration, registering and using data, and comprehension. Within these aspects, we see the Transpersonal Pattern: dispersion.

Anxiety and self-centeredness can create Heat and Dampness. Substances accumulate, and the mind becomes even dimmer.

It is difficult for the Cerato person to process, at both the digestive and mental levels. So nutrients and information are poorly used.

Virtues

The internal point of reference with which the Cerato person does not quite succeed in connecting lies in the Water element. She is the seat of Wisdom, of that which lies in the deepest part of self, in other words, in contact with the transcendental and universal aspect. The inexhaustible source.

In order to get down there, the light of Fire—the Heart's consciousness—is needed. Without it, there is no seeing or hearing anything.

The painting teacher, Roberto Bosco, would say to his students with Cerato characteristics, "You're sitting on a chest full of gold coins, and you can't manage to take one out to buy yourself a lowly sandwich," referring to someone replete with resources that he doesn't know he has, and so he doesn't use them.

Comments

The Cerato person doesn't manage to nourish herself from her interior, but nor is it possible to do so with what comes from outside. She underestimates her own wealth, stuffing herself with whatever she can get through asking this or that source. Even so, nothing satiates. The only thing that will fill her is to eat and drink from her own wellspring. As Ricardo comments, Heather is a very appropriate essence.

Some of the disorders present in this personality evoke what in Chinese Medicine we call Wind, whose characteristics are constant Movement and change, dispersion and the unforeseeable. This Flower Essence allows us to approach all sorts of changing and migratory symptoms: nonlocalized illnesses and those that change quickly. Restlessness, tics, tremors, dizziness. Also in colds, flu, and allergies—imbalances related to external influences—to which the Cerato type is very susceptible.

Centaury

Organs, Emotions, Psyche

The Kidney

If we look, according to the plant's signature, at the type of soil in which Centaury buries its roots, we can understand what kind of environment nourished the Centaury personality: short on affection but compact, in other words, with no room for individuality. An environment of emotional poverty and poor development of the individuation process (we'll see this in relation to Water and Wood). So Centaury goes unnoticed, blending in with the environment. Its strong roots are capable of penetrating these soils; somehow this type carries within itself the Virtues necessary for carrying out the struggle, in order to learn.

The Centaury type seeks to avoid conflict, confrontation, and placing boundaries. How does she do this? By appealing to an imbalanced Water force: docile, changeable, flexible for others to form her and shape her according to their whim. Ready to take the indicated form, she has no qualms with wearing dresses of humiliation. This is the point at which her intention to go unnoticed is truncated; the magnitude of her submission and malleability calls the attention of the casual observer. If she were to use this fluidity on herself, she would quickly learn her lesson.

The Kidney's Psyche bestows capacities allowing the Centaury person to have at her disposal the strength, direction, and elements necessary to change.

Centaury Flower Essence strengthens the Kidney. Toning this Organ by any other means known will help the Flower Essence's action.

Strengthening the Kidney's basic qualities will, for starters, put the person in a condition to exercise a stronger will; this will be the engine allowing other aspects to manifest themselves. She will have at her disposal a more well-defined sense of her own authority and internally perceived prospects for self-affirmation, all accompanied by a growth in determination.

When the Kidney is more firm, the qualities bestowed by its Psyche begin working effortlessly, becoming spontaneous, in accordance with Dr. Bach's proposal to not fight against defects.

When there is a pronounced deficiency in Water's Energy, there is a tendency toward self-destruction. Before reaching this point, the person may pass through Olive, Mustard, and Wild Rose states. Not awakening qualities that lie in wait in Water keeps the person fearful, in submission, unable to use will to oppose adversity or the wills of others, and the person experiences anxiety, angst, even total apathy, particularly in taking full control of her own life's direction.

Curiously, it is the Kidney that gives origin to and nourishes the bones, which give structure, solidity, and defense (among other things) to our bodies. Some of the difficulties that the Centaury type may present are: bone disorders, weakness in the lumbar area and the knees, ringing in the ears, growth disturbances (it is hard for them to grow, to be independent), general weakness (most of all as constitutional Kidney deficiency), and reduced immunity.

The Flower Essence provides Energy. It supports Defensive Energy's action, which protects the surface of our body from changes in the weather. It allows us to adapt and to defend ourselves efficiently, and I sustain that this is even true in the case of inclement emotional weather in the environment (Walnut Essence intervenes in the task).

Centaury Essence is an important helper in any change, given that a high quantity and quality of Energy is needed to make change.

The Centaury person's behavior erodes his vital strength and does so in pursuit of any path but his own.

The fuel for carrying out one's life plan is stored in the Kidney. This potential is freed up when we are following our own path, when we are, as Dr. Bach would say, the captains of our own ship. When this is not the case, we do not have access to this energetic "quantum."

The Liver

We know that when taking the Flower Essence, anger and aggression are, simply put, a frequented station on the road toward the Virtues, demonstrating that the person has arrived at Wood's territory whose rebalancing is indispensable. It constitutes the first Movement toward delimiting one's own space. But rather than drawing it with calm, firm authority, the uncontrolled fury of so many unspoken words is needed.

It is a first and imperfect balancing act; up till now, Wood's balanced Energy went underexpressed with things unsaid, fear and timidity, and want for one's own desires and projects.

When the Centaury type begins taking charge of herself, she must learn to organize daily life and recognize her own desires. Anger breathes life into the strength and enthusiasm she was missing for digging in her heels, reaching down into her roots, and saying, "Here I am, and if you want to cross this line, you had better well ask my permission."

Of course, we'll find it rather startling to see this person—who a few days ago was docile, benevolent, and empathetic to the point of disappearing into others, who spoke rather softly, and who was easy prey to the point that she seemed dim witted, blind—suddenly become robust, impulsive, and even indignant in the face of others' attempts at directing her. The authority and determination gained through strengthening the Kidney are used, at first, with fury and reclamation.

We might take into consideration the state of the Gallbladder, which, as we mentioned in the section on Cerato, provides the courage to act to bring about change despite psychological pressure and fear. Weakness in this Viscera makes the person shy, fearful, and easily discouraged.

Virtues

Centaury's lesson in the Virtues is about coming into the possession of a wiser and more intelligent kind of benevolence: the Virtues of Water and Wood brought into a balance for serving one's own mission and for serving others.

Through its Psyche, the Kidney provides the will to live regarding one's own life purpose along with the strength and Energy necessary for bringing this purpose to fruition.

Scleranthus

Scleranthus, along with Cerato and Cherry Plum, treats aspects of Wind, an element that generates a great deal of chaos.

Some characteristics of Wind are:

- It appears quickly.
- It is unpredictable.
- It diminishes coordination.
- It upsets the capacity for Movement, which can be chaotic or can end in paralysis.
- It changes the direction and position of things.
- It generates instability, imbalance, and apprehension.

Wind is observable in the Scleranthus type's chaotic, accelerated, and erratic thoughts that jump from one option to another. Likewise, we see Wind in the Scleranthus personality's emotional instability—its roller-coaster ups and downs.

Scleranthus Flower Essence acts on some of the Wind disorders that are related to instability and to a lack of control and coordination:

- Vertigo, fainting, spasms, trembling, tics, convulsions, uncoordinated movements, stiffness, paralysis
- Trembling or agitated hands, feet, and head; tongue spasms or trembling
- Migratory pain that appears and disappears
- Itching, burning, contraction, and unpleasant sensations in the skin and muscles
- Cramps or stiffness in the skin, nerves, blood vessels, muscles, Viscera
- Strokes
- Hemiplegia, facial paralysis
- Skin conditions that appear and disappear
- Stiff neck
- Hypertension

There is an obvious need for an anchor, a point of reference, to prevent Wind from sending everything flying off in all directions. We can find this anchor in the balanced functioning of the various Organs.

Organs, Emotions, Psyche

The Liver

When in harmony, this Organ prevents excesses, so it is important to balance Liver-related Emotions when treating Scleranthus-type problems. Mood swings are a clear sign of the failure of one of the important functions of the Liver.

This Organ relates very much with Wind; its dysfunctions generate Wind effortlessly, and likewise, Wind easily affects it.

When the Liver is in good working order, it provides the capacity to be resolute and decisive. It allows one to give organization and a clear meaning to life (Wind is disorganization). Difficulty with assertion and decisions generates frustration, disorientation, and apprehension, all of which can deviate toward anger.

Scleranthus Essence is a true helper in organizing one's life as it harmonizes rhythms, provides coordination, and balances and clears the mind. It gives stability, resolution, consistency, and concentration. Scleranthus Essence acts in favor of a balanced Liver, putting instinctive intelligence back into play.

Gallbladder

The Energy provided by the Gallbladder allows us to make decisions without becoming sidetracked by any sort of psychological pressure, and it facilitates the ability to make judgments. Working harmoniously, the Gallbladder increases determination.

The Heart

The Heart controls the equilibrium of all functions, including those of the psyche; the harmonious functioning and coordination of the totality of the person depend upon the Heart.

We would be wise to pay attention to Emotions that are related to the Organs that are implicated in Scleranthus states. By regulating those Emotions, we help the action of the Scleranthus Flower Essence.

Virtues

The Kidney provides the firm root that prevents Wind from sending the Scleranthus-type person off flying, thus the mind becomes centered without getting sidetracked, and the personality ceases to be vacillating and indecisive.

Comments

The constant examination and analysis of various options seriously wears the mind, and this use of Fire drains a huge amount of Energy and Essence.

The brain, hyperactive, uses up an important part of available Energy, in detriment to processes that repair the body, causing health to recede.

The Spleen also suffers the consequences of excess deliberation, upsetting its ability to provide nutrients, Blood, and Energy; it has to give up all its Energy to the mind's concentration.

Water Violet

Organs, Emotions, Psyche

The Lung

The Lung, through its Psyche, extends the veil that makes us feel like individual beings. It is the force that impels the desire to live for oneself, separate from others. We need this illusion in order to experience life as humans.

Water Violet persons present the paradox of having this force be so powerful and creating such a sense of separation that in the end it becomes self-sufficiency, ultimately invalidating the possibility for living a wide range of human experiences. It would seem that Water Violet takes the role of "being an individual" too seriously, entering fully into the isolation that is referred to in the Transpersonal Pattern.

Water Violet people feel the need to live in an environment that is as well defined as their individuality. And this is how they come up against various obstacles. They isolate themselves and encounter a certain balance there, an internal peace and harmony that makes them feel quite well. They settle fully into solitude. Any person, situation, or Emotion that trespasses this domain makes them feel uncomfortable, bothering them.

But harmony lived in isolation is only half of harmony. The other half is missing, the more complicated kind, the kind that can live within the world and with various types of people. I am tempted to say that a balance that needs isolation as a defense is a balance constructed of props.

We see it in the plant's signature: if it leaves the aseptic environment that it knows, its great fragility becomes obvious.

Although Water Violet persons can carry out a life in perfect solitude, enjoying the gifts they've been given, a problem difficult to resolve still remains: we come into this world to manifest certain potentials, and developing them requires contact with others. The person might be the most capable and self-sufficient person in the world, but it is within community and interaction with others that these capacities take on meaning.

Things don't really depend on him as much as he thinks. He arrived at a place where things were already constructed. The food he eats? The clothes he wears? The teachers who taught him? The books he read? The long line of humans who gave their bones up to experiencing the various ways of living on Earth? He got all of this and more without ever having to bat an eyelash.

It is in the Lung's realm, that of Metal (the element to which it belongs), where the issue of purity is at play. Both the Organ and the Large Intestine carry out the function of purifying the organism. Remember the plant's need for a clean space, free of contamination. As Jordi Cañellas points out, regarding its signature, the plant needs a habitat of extremely clean and quiet waters. The botanical family to which it belongs is rich in saponins, substances that are antiseptic and antibiotic.

Metal's terrain is a habitat of purity: that which can be shaped and hardened and maintain its form, that of rigor and hardness. This Energy has an important presence in Water Violet persons, and (as Ricardo tells us) these individuals have a tendency toward marked disorders in the cervical spine that can extend into the dorsal area where the lungs are found.

We generally know that rejection* is a trait present in Water Violet types, but looking at the plant's signature, shouldn't we also be talking

---

*[In reference to Beech —*Trans.*]

about Crab Apple? This essence might allow this type of person to get a little bit closer to his devalued fellow humans.

Sadness and grief are Emotions that impact the Lung, and constricting the chest influences the Heart who is likewise touched by a lack of joy. We might notice symptoms like shortness of breath, chest pressure, quiet voice, cough, general weakness, difficulty breathing, lethargy, weak appetite, palpitations.

The Kidney

We might think of Water Violet types as having overdeveloped Water qualities like authority, self-affirmation, determination, the capacity to stay solid on their path despite obstacles, and will. All of these are traits that allow for a life of solitude, but when just a bit off-balance they easily turn into stiffness, obstinacy, and pride.

A Customized World

Water Violet persons seek a custom-fit world with minute chances for visitors. We notice this in the environment in which the plant develops, being (as Jordi emphasizes) the only aquatic plant of the system. But water has other qualities that this personality could do well to cultivate.

In reference to its signature, when the plant is in flower, it releases its roots from the soil and lets itself float, carried by the current—an aspect more aligned with the Daoist image of water, which flows flexibly, freely, fearlessly, with great adaptability, coming into contact with whatever the flow offers. The rudder is whatever the current chooses from moment to moment (controlling the rudder of one's own life seems to be a combination of going with the flow, guiding the flow, and at the same time having a course and an intention).

Water makes no distinctions; it embraces everything and flows by always putting itself beneath, but its power is unstoppable. The antithesis of pride and rigidity.

Virtues

Clearly, as Ricardo expresses, the Water Violet type needs to cultivate various Virtues.

Benevolence, related to the Liver (as we've mentioned with other Flowers); integrity; reciprocity, related to the circulation and exchange of Energy between self and other, guaranteeing the integrity of both; and wisdom.

Comments

We have been using this essence for quite a while now to provide yin. It collaborates in adjusting Heat-related conditions where there is a yin deficiency, along with other Flowers that act on Heat like Vervain, Impatiens, Agrimony, and Holly. Likewise, when there is dryness; Yin in this case means fluids and flexibility. We've observed that fluids have an important role with respect to rigidity and flexibility.

Gentian

Organs, Emotions, Psyche

A heavy portion of the imbalances present in the Gentian person's way of being are related to different aspects of the Spleen's and Lung's activities. We will take a look at some of the most important ones.

The Spleen

Part of intellectual functioning depends upon the Spleen, especially the kind we call logical thought: the capacity to think, to memorize, to organize and comprehend information. These qualities may be at our disposal when there is Energy and balance in this Organ.

These functions take a turn in the Gentian type, converting them into defects, into obstacles in learning and development. They become what Ricardo points out as "analysis that is critical, negative and almost always distorted from reality."

This is to say that an instrument that allows one to evaluate, classify, and comprehend knowledge for later use in daily life, and made particular by the angle of one's own life experience, loses its flexibility, tending to nullify its integration with other forms of knowing, such as intuition.

Direct perception—less obscured by logical and intellectual scaffolding, later to be integrated through comprehension and classification by analysis—in the Gentian type is opposed by a previous structure in perception. Here is the root of rigidity: this previous structure is the Gentian type's negative, pessimistic view of the world. No matter what is happening, the Gentian person tends to superimpose this matrix, making the world fit into it.

This happens, in part, for want of development of the Spleen's Virtues, confidence and faith, which would allow the person to change the a priori vision she has of the world and construct a new, more appropriate, less partial matrix. A more integral and all-encompassing view. Clearly, understanding yin and yang's opposition, alternation and permanent change, is not one of the Gentian person's priorities. Facing a lack of faith and confidence, the critical and analytical side grows out of proportion, giving rise to worry, which drains the Spleen's Energy.

The Lung
Let's look at the Emotions frequently found in the Gentian personality and which may affect the Lung: pessimism, dejection, dismay, Emotions that can lead to depression (and let's remember that these Emotions can just as much affect the Lung as be a consequence of imbalances in this Organ's functioning). Once we've verified Lung-related disorders, serious vulnerability will also become apparent, in consonance with the Transpersonal Pattern—fragility—as well as a marked difficulty in adapting to change, especially changes that pose difficulties.

Being as it is that the Lung's activities allow us to incorporate the new and throw out the old, as it is said in Chinese Medicine, this balance may be injured given that the Gentian person doesn't allow much space for that which is new—another facet of difficulty with change. A poorly functioning Lung doesn't support the incorporation of creative resources for sustaining change nor for feeling motivated, "with wind in one's sails."

When the Lung's Psyche is imbalanced, we may observe in Gentian persons a propensity for jealousy, a desire to abandon everything, and disinterest.

Breathing may be an indicator that a person has some real Gentian components. The inhalation may be short and/or quick, shallow, or there may be other respiratory troubles.

The Lung and Spleen have vital importance (once we've been born into the world) in nutrition and in learning. Chances for obtaining resources that support us and allow us to feel prepared for facing life are determined, in part, by these Organs. Also the capacity to unpack and assimilate our experiences. Likewise, an adequate supply of Blood and Energy depend upon their proper functioning, which, when diminished, determines weakness and reduced defenses—this is to say, greater vulnerability in every sense, less Energy available for the processes of learning and change, less circulation of nutrients and of information.

Disorders may present themselves in two big areas, digestion and breathing, resulting in illnesses that could be a consequence of imbalances in these functions.

The Kidney
Willpower is not one of Gentian's outstanding Virtues. Any possibility for increasing it will be beneficial. The same thing goes for tenacity and the strength to stay true to one's goals without abandoning them at the first sight of obstacles.

The Gallbladder
The Gallbladder helps the Kidney, providing resistance when facing psychological pressure. It helps one to have more determination and assertion, to not become so easily discouraged.

Virtues
Virtues related to Gentian are confidence and faith, as mentioned, in relation to the Spleen, and rectitude, the cultivation of which supports the Lung and which refers to one's attitude facing losses and gains, the balance between accumulation and release.

Comments
Observing the plant's signature and looking at the item Jordi exposes about the ecology of the species, we see that it "grows in dry fields, sometimes in very poor soils," which is to say that its preexisting environment is not very "nourishing." Taking into account that, when talking about the Spleen and Lung we mentioned that there could be failure in nourishing, we might consider that in the Gentian type there has been a lack of affection in the emotional terrain from the start; a malnourishment in substance and Emotion that could lead the person to have a pessimistic, negative view of the world, to expect less, not more; an environment where confidence, faith, and hope don't have much place, and

there is nothing to do but to continue experiencing the worst. This can probably explain in part why Gentian is slow to change and to learn.

Rock Rose

Organs, Emotions. Psyche

The description for this personality type speaks of someone who is sensitive, labile, delicate, and very skittish. In short, someone vulnerable who gives the sensation that he is perceiving more than just a simple fork dropped or having been called on by someone when he wasn't paying attention. Things like this startle the Rock Rose type in an extreme way. It's as if these events abruptly penetrated his perceptual field, without any resistance, going straight to his Heart. As if he had not enough time or instruments to decant stimulus and turn it into something routine. Something like having his nervous system open and raw, denied of all filters and defenses.

From the Chinese Medicine viewpoint, we find situations in which it is possible for people to exhibit traits of this personality.

The Gallbladder

This Viscera, besides carrying out digestive functions, has certain traits that make it a special Viscera. One of these traits is that its balance depends on bravery—the courage available to us. It provides us with fortitude for facing emotional pressures that come from our environment, creating, in a sense, part of our defensive capacity.

When the Gallbladder is weak, whether it's due to one's constitution or to some disorder, the person becomes very vulnerable and is easily startled; even sleep may be fragile, the person awakening with a start. There is great shyness and lack of courage. The person finds it hard to stand his ground and mark his territory and may possibly have difficulty making decisions.

The Heart

Deficiencies in the Heart, especially in its Blood, also leave the person rather defenseless; she gets frightened and startled. The mind cannot settle, and the person is overcome with the above-mentioned disorders.

On occasion, Gallbladder and Heart deficiencies are presented together. It may also be a constitutional weakness of both Organs.

Sudden, potent, and paralyzing fear affects the Heart, generating symptoms like palpitations, insomnia, a fainting sensation, loss of mental clarity, and others. The disorganization generated by panic is due in part to the Heart's responsibility for the functional coherency of the whole organism, for the Heart is Emperor.

The Lung
The Lung also participates in this process given that its debility can generate vulnerability and scarce capacity for adapting to changes. Moreover, the Lung defends us from things coming from the environment.

The Kidney
The Kidney is affected in practically every type of fear. Its Psyche sustains the mind in a way that allows one to remain calm when facing panic situations.

Sudden fear drains and disorganizes Energy. And it is the Kidney who will have to face the situation, providing Essence.

Virtues
Each one of the Organs mentioned supports the capacity for bravery, for having courage, the indispensable courage needed for existing in the world.

Comments
Deficient Liver Blood may lead to serious fear states.

Pain due to Blood stagnation and perceived as piercing, and also that which is produced by cold (both are very intense), may be approached using this Flower Essence.

The essence may be used to alleviate general hypersensitivity, assisting Flowers like Chicory, Beech, and Holly, among others.

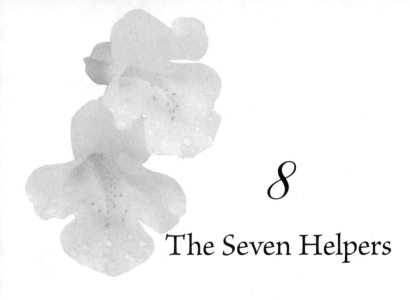

8

The Seven Helpers

Gorse

*B*lood and Energy deficiencies as well as a lack in vital spiritual strength can produce Gorse states. But what may also happen is that when desperation, surrender, and resignation set in—all descriptive of the attitude that Gorse Essence treats—Blood and Energy production systems deteriorate, creating a situation that anchors and reinforces the symptoms.

Adaptation to Change and the Lung Psyche's Dissolving Force

The Lung

Many of the Emotions and mental states that afflict persons experiencing Gorse states create imbalance in the Lung. Pessimism and a negative projection of the future generate disturbances in the Lung's capacity to produce and command Energy. The pessimistic attitude may be accompanied by a fear of the future (an imbalance in this Organ's Psyche) adding emotional nuances to the Gorse state.

The capacity for adapting to change clearly has its limits, and these present many varied forms in different people, consistent with other factors such as the strength available for tolerating frustration, among other factors.

The Lung's Psyche provides us with the solvency necessary for adapting to change, but when this faculty is exaggerated, negativity and a desire to abandon emerge as the mind and heart become overrun with darkness. The need to surrender becomes imperious.

The destructive forces of the Lung's Psyche, which tend toward dissolution, have been activated. These pull toward separation, toward becoming reclusive within the thin margins of oneself. They favor crystallization and a return to the material aspect of being, to earth. They pull the person toward death. To give up or remain on the sidelines of the flow of events is one form of death. It also leaves he who suffers from this state disengaged from his destiny.

Depending on the depth and breadth of the Gorse state, the pull toward death may span from a simple period of desperation and of stepping offstage to heal one's wounds, to an actual abandonment of life.

The strength of the Heart's Psyche is what can balance the dissolving pull of the Lung's Psyche. As we'll see further ahead, the Kidney's Psyche adds support to the Heart's intentions. If signs of deterioration in the area of influence of this last Organ appear, treatment may be more difficult.

The Lung also participates in a facet of immunity (Defensive Energy), which protects us while allowing us to adapt to the environment. In Gorse states, immunity loses support given that immunity is not only about fighting but also about adapting to the environment and achieving a state of harmony with it.

The surrender of one's capacity to adapt brings stiffness. It is in this sense that, for supporting the action of Gorse Flower Essence, it could be very favorable to give Star-of-Bethlehem, an essence that supports flexibility, the reconnection of energetic circuitry, and the treatment of underlying trauma. And by now it surely escapes no one that Walnut is another auxiliary essence that can help Gorse Essence on its mission, positively influencing the feeling of condemnation brought on by the knowledge of having a disorder cataloged as hereditary, as Ricardo mentions. It also supports the capacity to flow with change.

The Kidney

Taking Gorse Essence appears to ward off the Lung Psyche's destructive demons, but there is another area where the Gorse drama might unfold, and this is in the Kidney.

People with weak Kidney constitution experience a diminished capacity for fighting and persisting, as well as weakened immunity and physical strength. They are more vulnerable to the blows of adversity. Their will to live is weakened. This situation could clearly be the root of various other floral states like Mimulus, Larch, Centaury, to name a few. In the section on Olive, we will look at things again from this perspective.

As we've mentioned with other Flowers, chronic illness demands a lot of the Kidney, and this is how a Gorse state may arise, deepen, or feed off itself. When this Organ's Energy has a marked deficiency, the person may enter into a deep Gorse state, while a less pronounced deficiency creates conditions for a predisposition to experience Gorse in varying degrees of intensity.

The Kidney participates directly in resistance to illness, so when it is affected, immunity is notably weakened.

The strength of the Kidney's Psyche, manifesting itself as the will to live, opposes the destructive forces at work when the Lung's Psyche is out of balance.

Some symptoms that give us signs of Kidney disorders are weakness in the lumbar area and the knees, memory lapses, early aging, auditory or tooth disorders, accumulation of fluids, and problems in reproductive capacities, among others.

The Spleen

Want for faith and confidence, at times unconscious, can undermine the Spleen's ability to metabolize foods and extract from them their most subtle components. At first, this may show up as a slight abdominal discomfort, especially after eating. Little by little it will grow to the point of abdominal swelling and distention following meals. There may be tiredness and an appearance of symptoms like reduced appetite and a feeling that the limbs are weaker than usual.

Following this, one might notice soft stools and that a pale yellow tinge to the skin begins to appear, which in this case describes mucus and fluid accumulation. On occasion there is also insomnia and palpitations, and a degree of anxiety may arise.

A reduced wealth of personal faith is not the only thing that can generate these symptoms, but when they exist, and more so when they are chronic, we must keep this possibility in mind and move from the physical symptoms to deduce the Virtues that may be in question.

Another route that disorders may take is that of upsetting intellectual capacity. There will then be diminished concentration and attention, foggy thoughts, difficulty studying, and no abundance of ideas.

Blood and Energy give the mind a base for adequately developing itself. The Spleen is an extremely important Organ as much in the production of Blood and Energy as in its distribution to the whole body.

Impulse and the Capacity to Fight

If the Spleen and Lung are damaged, the ability to generate Blood and Energy are affected and can create, as a consequence, a tendency to lack impulse, strength, and the capacity to fight. This tendency will deepen if the Kidney is also weak.

Nevertheless, the plant's signature shows us that its capacities for regeneration and regrowth are far from negligible. Its roots go deep. This is how taking the Flower Essence can help to strengthen Kidney Energy so that it can work on regenerating the body's substrates and tissues as well as renovate and sustain life.

Once the ability to adapt to change has been recovered—overcoming the Lung Psyche's destructive tendencies—and the Kidney has been fortified, the conditions for relaunching an invigorating cycle have been created. A base has been established that will allow the explosive force of the Liver to bud out in something that was believed to be dead.

Gorse Flower Essence stimulates the whole life cycle.

Comments

It would make sense to ask ourselves what situation a Gorse person finds herself in with respect to manifesting her life's purpose. It could be that difficulties in accomplishing her purpose lead to a state of desperation and surrender, or, on the contrary, that an inability to get in touch with her own path has stripped life of its meaning, and, finding no meaning in the tasks of living, she is overcome with a Gorse state. And so it becomes important to take into account that we might also need to treat this existential issue with the help of Wild Oat, among other essences.

Considering what Jordi has said about the signature, one form of supporting the Flower's action may be to encourage the person to do things with others, to carry out some task that interests her, and, more than for her own benefit, that it be a way of preparing the terrain for others' development. The impasse or abandon that the Gorse state implicates in the attainment of one's path, one's destiny, might be remedied by remembering that fulfilling one's destiny occurs with others and based on manifestations that imply the creation of something favorable to others.

The Transpersonal Pattern—and experience using the essence in this sense—indicate the Flower's usefulness in cases of Organ deficiency. An Organ may reach a state of Blood and/or Energy vacancy due to excess work (Oak), which can lead to a state of surrender (Gorse), which, furthermore, makes Olive Essence necessary. It is advisable to maintain the dosage of Oak, given that other Organs may have more demand placed on them (Elm), due to carrying part of the weight that the Organ in deficiency cannot carry.

Oak

The current way of life in modern society greatly facilitates Oak states. The proposition is to work an infinite number of hours with very few rest periods, insufficient and inadequate time for meals, and sometimes with just a few hours of sleep. This lifestyle leads some people to Olive states, while other more resistant people sustain Oak states. Likewise, the contemporary social organizational model is a good refuge for these personalities.

It is important to keep in mind that, even in situations where Oak shows up as a personality trait, the person may have areas where he shows much less tension and more freedom. This disparity reinforces the dynamic view that Ricardo proposes for the Flowers, which allows for the existence of variances in subtlety and quality and permits an evaluation of the intensity and the depth of an Oak-related imbalance in each person.

Blood, Energy, and Structure

The Oak type's lifestyle is, quite simply, a factor generating pathology. It exhausts Blood, Energy, and various tissues and body parts, depending on the type of overexertion.

We'll take a general look at how we might manage dysfunctions triggered by this state.

If one submits oneself to predominately physical wear and tear, the consequence will be the gradual exhaustion of Energy in various Organs, resulting in physical and mental weariness, weakness and/or weariness in the limbs, and over time dysfunctions will appear in Organs that have less constitutional strength.

Energy stagnation and distending pain may appear in the part of the body most used for the specific physical labor. Every type of activity has its area of impact, and traditionally it is said that standing for long periods of time affects the bones, while walking too much influences the tendons.

Muscles are Energy reserves for the internal Organs, so by fatiguing the muscles excessively and repeatedly, one ends up exhausting these Organs, and the consequences become increasingly more severe.

Excessive mental labor may bring on a reciprocal amount of digestive and sleep disorders, poor memory, heart palpitations, dizziness, various types of hemorrhaging, menstrual disturbances, and asthenia (abnormal weakness or lack of Energy).

Much time is spent seated when doing intellectual activity, and this damages muscles, overworks the eyes, exhausts the Blood, and affects the mind.

In some cases the overexertion is as much physical as it is mental. What complicates the situation is that a person in an Oak state doesn't perceive any of these signals, or doesn't pay them any attention, but rather subordinates all else to the fulfillment of duty.

It is even possible that, due to Oak's great strength, any of the disorders mentioned could take a while to appear. So the Oak type's physical and mental resistance turn out to be a weakness. Having no symptoms, or not noticing them, the activity and attitude extend over longer periods of time.

Long-Term Effects

There comes a point at which the daily intake of Energy—through foods, liquids, and Energy obtained from the air—no longer covers the needs of such intense daily activity. When Energy derived by the Spleen (from foods and liquids) and the Lung (from the air) is no longer enough, it is the Kidney that must suffer the loss of its Energy stores. When Kidney Energy begins to be depleted, weariness becomes much deeper. It will no longer be enough to sleep well, eat well, and get enough fresh air; recovery will take a lot longer.

The various ailments that were being carved out of years of physical, mental, and emotional rigor will finally make their appearance as pathologies that forbid the Oak person from further depleting his resources: severe illnesses, hypertensive crisis, heart disease, or serious exhaustion.

The following Organs may be particularly affected due to the peculiarities of Oak states.

The Lung

The Lung is related with the physical body's capacity to *feel,* to perceive sensations of Movement and the body's location in space, and also to perceive sensations stemming from muscles, Viscera, bones, and joints. All of these sensations and information—when the information that makes itself heard is interpreted by the Oak person as weakness and weariness—is persistently silenced. More fervently repressed are those sensations indicating the need to stop and take a break. A deaf ear is turned to these sensations, because to feel them and to interpret them would leave no other choice than to take into account the pains, the fatigue, the tension, the stiff muscles, the need for nourishment, and so on.

The ability to experience pleasure results, in part, from the capacities to feel the body, as mentioned above. To not perceive sensations produced by the body and to postpone pleasure, overemphasizing duty, are characteristics of Oak imbalances that foment disorders in the Lung and its sphere of influence.

The Kidney

Force of will, tenacity, physical strength, and persistence for achieving goals are all Virtues associated with the Kidney, one of the key Organs in an Oak state. Practicing these Virtues in an exaggerated and inflexible way turns them into defects. Chronic Oak states end up harming this Organ.

Sexual Energy is closely related with the Kidney, and it is this Energy that lets us feel pleasure, in a broad sense of the word. The continuous depletion of Kidney Energy notably diminishes the capacity to feel pleasure and chips away at part of the Essential Energy available for unfolding one's destiny.

People with Oak as a personality trait are unable to disobey mandates that they once upon a time received and subsequently took on as their own. As they continue, they deplete the strength and Energy that they were given for carrying out their own celestial mandate.

The will to live in service of one's own life purpose and unique path tends to get left by the wayside, leaving open and vulnerable a very sensitive Kidney-related area.

The Spleen

Oak situations tend to subject the Spleen to considerable pressure. As we've already mentioned, the Organ is forced to generate Blood and Energy at a rate not at all advisable. This important Organ becomes even further debilitated from the added impact of chronic worrying seen in Oak states.

Infusing the experiences of life into one's personality, as an essential part of learning, is one of the tasks of the Spleen's Psyche. Someone in an Oak state doesn't seem to dedicate much time or attention to this aspect of life. He would rather keep his head down and nose to the grindstone.

Disorders in the muscles and in deep tissues of vital importance, such as bones, bone marrow, the spinal cord, and brain tissue, should be kept in mind when working with persons who show long-standing Oak states.

Another Form of Malnourishment

A person in an Oak state submits himself to a serious type of malnourishment that is not usually seen as such. He doesn't let himself be nourished by affection as this is an area very difficult for him to manage. He doesn't enrich himself with music, theater, cinema, and so on. Art is not experienced as a way to nourish the soul and broaden one's horizons but rather as a totally superfluous activity lacking in any interest whatsoever. People in Oak states have a linear point of view; they don't exercise their peripheral vision much.

Comments

Ricardo comments that it is difficult for the person to express the tension that is generated by his Oak state. This situation leads to stagnation of Liver Energy and can generate more anger and anxiety, sustaining a cycle and mounting a pressure very difficult to manage if expressive outlets aren't found.

Taking Oak Flower Essence helps to avoid drainage of ancestral Energy amassed in the Kidney and reestablishes Energy provisioning, which thus opens a good pathway for recovering physical, emotional, and psychological sensitivity without losing strength, tenacity, and resistance. It's an appealing route too, letting wisdom (the Virtue of the Kidney) help the Oak person to develop her nobility, courage, and hope with better strategy and sensitivity, inspiring those around her.

The Flower Essence also favors the prevention of disorders in the Organs mentioned and in their areas of influence, and (following the Transpersonal Pattern), it helps relieve the Organ or Organs that find themselves working excessively to compensate for inadequate functioning of other Organs.

Heather

People in a Heather state truly have a great capacity for concentration; everything is swept up into their great tornado and funneled down to land at that central spot that is their frenzied need for affection—even though it may mean holding their company hostage.

This preoccupation with the self—the observation of the self in every little detail—comes out of emotional needs, but the act of being so attentive to oneself is in itself a mental effort. It is a focused concentration that if it were not so exaggerated and repetitive would be a Virtue.

But as it is, this mental focus stagnates. Energy follows the mind, and when the mind gets stuck in some aspect, Energy becomes stagnant and so do organic fluids.

We can understand, then, how mucus and phlegm begin to form and accumulate. In the same way that people in a Heather state are "sticky," the heaviness of their relations with others also has a correlation in the body.

The stagnation that is produced by focusing both mind and intention on one's own self and own happenings slows down the functioning of the Liver, which is the Organ in charge of keeping things flowing at a regular and appropriate rhythm. The resulting obstruction, besides producing various substances in the body, predisposes the person in a Heather state to anger and explosiveness, as well as animosity in interpersonal relations, as Ricardo mentions.

The Spleen

Depending on the virulence and duration of the Heather state, we may observe a range of symptoms, from a simple and passing slowness in the circulation of Energy to the accumulation of very thick mucus, the formation of nodules, and more serious deterioration of the functioning of the Spleen and other Organs that help metabolize liquids.

This mental-physical circuit guarantees a chronic state; internal stagnation fosters obsession and preoccupation, detaining thoughts by keeping them stuck in the same pathways without arriving at anything new. The mind loses clarity. It also becomes increasingly difficult to establish relationships.

The Spleen's Psyche carries out the important function of "maintaining the Integrity of the Individual" (Jarret, mentioned in Alexander, "Nutrindo a vitalidade"). In Heather states, this function is exaggerated and is carried out in a way that stagnates, probably as a consequence of the emptiness felt by the Heather person. This leads him to compensate by retaining, accumulating. Heather Flower Essence overlaps in various ways with Chicory, whose action is quite complementary to Heather's. In both personalities there is a dissociation that, in extreme cases, can lead to excision mechanisms nearing psychosis.

The Spleen's Psyche, mentioned above, is associated with another function, that of reciprocity, through which life force is regulated in order to maintain a balance between the person and the world, with the goal of sustaining one's own subsistence while also enabling a balanced exchange. The Heather person evidently seeks a totally asymmetrical and unidirectional exchange with the world, toward oneself, "all for me."

Angst and a feeling of emptiness prevent the Heather person from perceiving that if she were less self-centered and less insistent, this very emptiness would tend to fill itself naturally. The act of retaining and of permanently trying to satiate herself stops up any chances of actually getting what she needs.

Accumulation

The person in a Heather state fills up on heavy, dense, turbid substances but still feels empty of affection, with a voracious, interminable need. In the body, it is quite clear that what remains when one cannot "let go" are waste products; what ought to be shed fills the space of what is really needed.

This brings us to the topic of lack of selectivity. Heather personalities are not concerned about who it is keeping them company; they're so busy with their own concerns that they don't discriminate between what nourishes and what does not. All this lack of discrimination is implicated in present or future disorders in the Small Intestine (keep in mind the Small Intestine's relationship with the Heart).

Symptoms of accumulation can be found

- in the muscles
- in the chest and abdomen, with a "full" sensation, of pressure and distension
- as a feeling of heaviness in the head
- in the limbs and in the body in general (a heavy feeling from which the mind doesn't escape)
- as obstructed digestion
- as disturbances in the elimination of urine and feces
- as leukorrhea
- in some types of rheumatism
- in the skin, as festering eruptions and as other symptoms

The Heart

Heat may be generated as a consequence of Energy's prolonged stagnation due to the Heather person's anxiety and food intake (often greasy and spicy foods), intensifying "chronicity" as a factor in this state. Speech also becomes accelerated and excessive due to Heat.

Heat affects the Heart, which was already getting overworked from excessive reflection, manifested in Heather states as self-involvement, which creates more mental agitation, anxiety, angst, and hyperemotiveness, possibly leading to a state of confusion.

The Virtue related to the Heart's Psyche is propriety, having to do with the capacity to adjust one's actions within a social context and implying a certain consciousness of the environment and sense of what is appropriate.

The Lung

The Lung is one of the places mucus tends to get deposited. Dysfunctions in this Organ can magnify egocentric tendencies. Thanks to the Lung's Psyche, we have a strong enough sensation of being separate from the whole that we are able to perceive ourselves as individual entities and carry out the human experience. In Heather states, it is possible that the sensation of separateness is too intense, that somehow the person got more anchored in this particular aspect of being an individual than other facets of the individual human experience. Heather-type persons, by invading others' personal space, even through speech, are trying to recover a perception of unity with others and to belong to the whole; they are seeking union through a demand for attention and Energy. Such are the sensations of separation and panic that a person in this state is begging, "come to me all the time and always."

Resolving the paradox of being with others, in community, in order to constitute oneself as an individual isn't simple for anyone and can become an unresolvable problem for the Heather type. Freedom and independence are closely related to the capacity to feel oneself as part of the whole and to make a personal contribution in relation to one's life purpose.

Viewed from another angle, we might see that the Heather person needs to develop rectitude (the Virtue related to the Lung's

Psyche), which allows us to find a balance between what we accumulate and what we eliminate. Considering that the way the Heather person behaves in the world is very much related to aspects of the Lung, it is important to keep in mind disorders in this Organ and its areas of influence so that we may follow the case with an idea of a prognosis.

Comments

In a Heather state, angst and neediness shroud everything, making it difficult for one to connect with one's potential and life purpose. Once again, connecting with one's own path is of vital importance. This in itself sparks one to do things that benefit not only oneself but also influence the community. Let's say it one more time: evolution is something we do together.

Organs of elimination may be particularly affected (skin, Large Intestine, Kidney, Lung, respiratory mucus, saliva glands, vaginal mucus, Liver), given that in the Heather state the force of contraction is powerful, moving in a direction contrary to the capacity to eliminate.

This force of contraction and inability to eliminate—related to sluggish circulation of Energy and fluids and the accumulation of phlegm and mucus—favor the acidification of the organism, provoking demineralization and other disorders. This situation is also present in any chronic illness.

Heather and Agrimony are possibly the two mental states affecting the most Organs and processes and are thus essences of great utility for preventing chronic degenerative illness.

It is interesting to confirm that certain Flower Remedies help to metabolize liquids, to liquefy mucus, and to eliminate it. Up in front we have Chicory, Heather, Willow, and Crab Apple; closely following are White Chestnut, Red Chestnut, and, in more general terms, Chestnut Bud.

Note also that some of the Heather plant's medicinal properties favor the elimination of Dampness, helping regulate the metabolism of liquids.

Rock Water

Water and Stone

Water and mountain are inseparable in Chinese painting. They give each other meaning and identity. Truly, they represent the two poles of the visible world and of universal transformation.

In order for this relationship to not be rigid, it needs mystery, the void, the unfathomable and impenetrable, that which is difficult to understand and impossible to control (and that with which the Rock Water type doesn't want to get too involved). If this aspect is accepted, water can have the firmness of a mountain, and stone the flexibility and fluidity of water.*

The Lung

When we use rigidity as a means for cultivating rectitude, the Virtue of this Organ becomes perverse. Ultimately, rectitude is no longer rectitude but rather a statute of hardness. If anything moves under this structure, there is danger of collapse, so (apparently) the only choice is to maintain the rigorous framework. And it is achieved at the expense of much Energy and repression. The exercise of rectitude converted into hardness is a structure created for protecting fragility.

A great part of our ability to adapt to change—something the Rock Water state is not very apt for—resides in the Lung's Psyche. Likewise, the Lung's Psyche makes it possible to have body consciousness and sensuality, to feel in the body that which comes from the environment, to feel through the skin. All these things the Rock Water type keeps at bay, or just simply represses with no awareness of them whatsoever.

Rock Water nonetheless cultivates a different aspect of the Lung and its Virtue, which is rectitude. But an imbalanced aspect—an excessive desire for perfection, to accumulate merit.

Metal's Energy of contraction balances Wood's Energy of expansion, but in Rock Water types, contraction is such that it detains and stagnates. Disorders related to fluids and Blood may present as stagnation (accumulation of substances) and dryness. Seriousness, order,

---

*For further reading about water and mountain, see François Cheng's book *Empty and Full: The Language of Chinese Painting*.

balance in the work rhythm, the notion of justice and discipline—all characteristics of Metal—become instruments for reining in authentic impulses (which are of course expressed disjointedly). They become instruments that isolate and separate.

Fluids have a marked relationship with physical flexibility. When fluids are diminished, one has difficulty moving and a tendency toward stiffness. Dryness, in this state, can also be observed as a poor capacity for creative response—a handcuffed and poor imagination.

Dryness draws our attention to fragility. As Ricardo mentions, dryness and hardness usually mask insecurity, fear, and a fragility that cannot survive even minimal disorder or change. Symptoms like dry hair, wrinkled or flaky skin, cracked eyes, scanty urine, dry stools, constipation, thirst, anxiety, insomnia, and some types of depression, among other symptoms, may be present.

Dryness also has an astringent effect that contracts. Irritation and Heat may arise, leading to various Flower states, among them, Beech.

The Liver

The iron fist that characterizes the Rock Water type injures the Liver's activity early on, generating initial stagnation in this Organ that, over time, will slow the circulation of both Energy and Blood, giving rise to internal Heat. From this situation a multiplicity of symptoms derive that may range from the appearance of cysts, tumors, various pains, and digestive disorders to vertigo, ringing in the ears, and migraines. In the emotional sphere, the process described is the base for orneriness and a petri dish for resentment. It is also another way to generate rigidity, observable in a loss of physical flexibility and a hardness in the muscles.

Benevolence—the Virtue corresponding to the Liver's Psyche—can, through its cultivation, help the Rock Water person, given that it urges us to include others in the development of our life's plan but without blocking the simultaneous unfolding of the paths of others.

Another aspect we may see in people who excessively restrict and control themselves is a loss of fluids: Blood, sweat, diarrhea, vomit, semen, urine. When there isn't authentic balance, what is controlled on one side is lost out the other.

We use Rock Water Essence along with Water Violet for treating Heat—especially Heat due to yin deficiency—when we need to reposition organic fluids after hemorrhages, diarrhea, vomiting, excessive sweating, and so on and in any dryness disorder. Walnut Essence can help with said liquid loss, while Rock Water Essence helps by working at the base of the energetic mechanisms that guarantee fluid and Energy circulation, averting stagnation.

The Kidney

The Rock Water type believes that to achieve Water's Virtue (wisdom) he must reduce his life to a point where there is no Movement or change. It's the old maneuver of trying to direct water's flow. He confuses excessive control with depth. He needs the depth of Water, not the exaggerated contraction of Metal.

Freezing Water's Psyche is another way he constructs rigidity: willpower and goal achievement carried out with a hardness devoid of any flexibility and with a tenacity bordering on insanity. What is more, what is being pursued with such obstinacy is an imposition of his narrow view of the world and, as such, is an action that does not correspond with his internal nature.

In this regard, Dr. Bach says, "They want to plan the world according to their own outlook instead of quietly and gently doing a little in the Great Plan" (*Twelve Healers and Four Helpers*).

In Daoist terms, it is an issue of wanting to administrate the world. The difficulty that Rock Water types have in this sense is that they do not perceive nor understand that there exists a type of action, void of self and self-importance, that stems out of internal nature and that adapts to the person and the environment. This type of action brings satisfaction, is effortless, and self-adjusts spontaneously and harmoniously with the external environment. It also allows potentials in one's own internal nature to be put into play, and these are what are needed for turning their part of "the Great Plan" into a reality. This type of action in itself emanates a virtuous influence that touches the environment and others, positively transforming them.

Rock Water types cover up the ignorance they have of their internal nature with self-imposed rules and repression. They do not accept themselves, and as Ricardo mentions, they do not know themselves. So they follow an artificial path that they themselves draw and that does not lead them toward manifesting their destiny.

In the Kidney, in the impenetrable depths of Water (element to which this Organ belongs), sexual Energy is stored, which, as we've referenced on other occasions, is very closely linked to the potential for carrying out our destiny given that it is one of the fuels that impels us. It is the kind of Energy that allows us to feel pleasure, be it from a caress, a food, or a poem. In the Rock Water person, sexual Energy is severely repressed, and as such, the person takes paths that run alongside perversion. In these arid deserts, the precious fuel that sustains the capacity for feeling pleasure and for spiritual realization is evaporated. Once again, the severe control aimed at maintaining a straight line ends up generating serious losses.

Comments

The Kidney and Lung suffer the consequences of the Rock Water mental state. The Heart is constricted and is missing chances to express joy. The Spleen may be affected as a consequence of the personality's obsessive component, which also detains and stagnates.

Water that flows and that travels paths retains within it various viewpoints. It has crossed various landscapes, has seen changing skies, has intuited rocks in the dark depths of Earth. As Julian Barnard suggests in *Form and Function,* the water that is lost to the light of the face of Earth slipped from view toward the silent depths, to return free of memory. Being itself, without discontinuing its flow, it distilled its countless attributes.

Finally: Regulation is successful because firmness and flexibility are proportionate and firmness is centered. It will not do to persist in painful regulation because that way leads to exhaustion. But it is not I who says so; it is written in the *I Ching.*

Olive

The Impact on the Kidney

As we mentioned in Oak, over-extending one's strength (which varies from person to person according to his or her constitution), hard times that demand a great expenditure over a prolonged period of time, and chronic illness all erode Kidney Energy, thus affecting Essential Energy. Intellectual or physical labor that doesn't allow time for rest and regeneration provoke the same erosion. When this happens, something more than just rest is needed in order to feel well again.

The classical use of Olive Flower Essence reveals situations in which Essential Energy needed a helping hand because the Energy obtained from air and food wasn't enough to meet needs. The Kidney became damaged, with disorders appearing in the Psyche, Emotions, and related areas.

We'll find in the Olive state a submission to life's difficulties and a loss of interest in life. The desire to do tasks that at other times seemed exceedingly interesting is lost, even to the point of utter apathy. Clearly, willpower is at a very low level. The person does not have at her disposal enough strength to persist toward set goals; despondency quickly sets in.

Facing such a lack of resources and drive, indecision and instability become routine, increasing any preexisting anxiety and angst.

If, on top of the Olive state, fears are also present, treating them with the corresponding Flowers will be important given that regulating the mind in this regard will increase chances for a more speedy recovery.

In the Olive state, immune capacity is diminished, bones may become weak, legs and knees lose strength and may even tremble. There is intellectual weariness, and the person may present paralysis or reduced sensitivity in the lower limbs, disorders in reproductive and sexual potency, hearing impairment, ringing in the ears, and so on.

Many of these symptoms, added to a weakened lumbar spine and vertigo, are also present in situations of sexual exhaustion, constituting a greater number of Olive states than one might think.

Olive Essence's regenerative power is clear in the plant's signature, and as we've mentioned earlier, regeneration is one of the Kidney's important tasks.

In any case, when the deficit is serious, it is important to give plenty of attention to nutrition given that it has in itself a yin aspect (raw materials for regeneration) and a yang aspect (through nutrient metabolism one also obtains Energy). Respecting the natural sleep cycle in consonance with the seasons is an indispensible tool when approaching a severe Olive state. Cultivating physical and mental stillness through any effective available method will prove to be of great help.

By fortifying Kidney Energy, the root of the body and mind is toned. This supports more presence and activity here on Earth, with more possibilities for learning and for being up to the task in the here and now.

Comments

In general, worry, obsession, sadness, and grief can increase exhaustion; regulating said Emotions will help in treating chronic Olive states. The essence is of great utility in cases of depression given that fortifying one's roots provides an important base for treating this disorder.

Surgical extraction of the uterus can lead to Olive states in women who already have a certain degree of Kidney deficiency. It is possible to observe a relationship between uterine extraction, Kidney Energy debilitation, and a thyroid gland that begins to function below capacity. The symptoms that follow can also be improved with Olive.

Essential Energy amassed in the Kidneys powers the engine that propels us on the path of realizing our own life's purpose. It is probable that Olive helps release the Essential Energy, which becomes fully available when used for activities that are aligned with fulfilling our destiny and not contrary to our internal nature.

Reflecting on this Flower Essence, we come to an issue of utmost importance: What do we do with our available Energy? And the question that follows: What do we want more Energy for? We'll see that when we gain more Energy, we tend to use it for making the same mistakes more "energetically."

Along the lines of Ricardo's commentary on the subject, what can sometimes happen is that taking Olive Essence "cuts off our supply," and we are forced to rest and reconsider if maybe we aren't dilapidating our vital Energy in self-imposed pipe dreams coming out of societal conditioning or simply out of hedonism. Being forced to rest, having no more access to the energetic riches, is a way to detain drainage. This is very important because each person's potential is found in the Kidneys, where primary vitality is stored.

Other times, the effect of taking the essence favors a balanced and strategic use of Energy, because even though the tasks may be arduous, and the intensity and unfolding in how they are carried out just as arduous, they are appropriate for the experience needed in fulfilling one's life purpose.

Taking Olive Essence probably helps to reduce the expenditure of Essential Energy and to optimize the Energy obtained from food and air.

The Flower Essence is used in a wide range of disorders that stem from deficiency and weakness. Some examples of its application:

- Disorders related to old age (a base Flower for this stage of life)
- When one possesses a weak constitution by inheritance
- During and following chronic illness
- In exhaustion generated by excessive sexual activity
- When there are nutrient deficiencies, a very common situation in modern societies
- Following hemorrhages or Blood loss
- In women who have had multiple pregnancies

Vine

The Kidney

The Vine type manifests imbalances that show overdeveloped attributes associated with the Kidney's Psyche. The tenacity and strength of will that allow him to persevere without becoming sidetracked in pursuing his goals become obstinacy.

Self-confidence and intense self-affirmation may develop into boldness. The Vine type's natural sense of authority and lineage of leadership degrade into authoritarianism, tyranny, and love of power. Facets of the Water element like danger, solidity, coldness, and impenetrability come to the fore. This very excess impedes the Heart's Psyche from deploying appropriate moral conscience within the Vine person's actions. In this way, greed for power lays waste to everything, including joy and sentiments of love.

In many cases, the Vine type considers other people as objects for satisfying his own desires and carrying out his own plans. That is why he expects complete passivity and submission to his orders.

Rather than developing wisdom and prudence, Virtues associated with the Kidney, he replaces them with authoritarianism; the ability to observe, comprehend, and orient are supplanted with force, direction, and control of processes. As if the Vine person really knew what

Dao grants to each human being, he names himself administrator of the world, which he considers a stage where each person and situation exists for satisfying his needs, for adapting to his vision.

This attitude clearly detains the flow of events, generating various sorts of stagnation, pain, and hardening in the body.

Circulation disorders, both arterial and venous, are typical, implicating the Heart and Liver. There may be a tendency to accumulate fluids. But the stagnation also extends to Energy, with the appearance of distending pain that responds well to the Flower Essence.

When authority cannot be exercised, frustration increases stagnation. So if explosions of anger can be verified in the person, we'll want to regulate them to minimize the risk of a cerebrovascular accident.

In some cases the other pole of Water may manifest itself, observable in a certain type of fear, weak will, and angst. In more complex situations, the person may present depression, a loss of life's meaning, loss of mental capacities, early onset dementia, or insanity. This last symptom could become a refuge to which the person retreats when chances for brandishing power are lost. It may be an extreme form of resistance, of obstinacy—of not letting anyone twist his arm.

In less serious cases, we may note another form of ignoring reality: deafness, in various types and degrees.

In the body, this other pole of Water may be observed in weak, cold, and stiff lower limbs, lack of resistance, ringing in the ears, frequent urination, premature wrinkles, and lack of sexual vigor, among other symptoms.

Another observable type of resistance with intent to control, in situations where control is no longer possible by direct methods, is in presenting symptoms and disorders that are very difficult to treat and that are not resolved despite multiple treatments. They tend to happen following a family's decision regarding housing or another type of quotidian arrangement that the person in the Vine state cannot contradict via power. Through the creation of symptoms, the person has the whole family under her command; she intends to prove that no one is capable of curing or even alleviating her suffering.

The lumbar area and knees are regions tied to the Kidneys, so it is not too hard to see how these could have pain, stiffness, and a variety of disturbances, likewise the teeth and bones.

Continuing with these associations, we must keep in mind the possibility of a cerebrovascular accident (as we've already mentioned), nervous system disturbances, and disorders in the ovaries, testicles, anus, and urethra. Passing urine and feces may also be affected.

Helping Vine people find balance is a truly complex thing. Many factors enter into play, and there are very marked deficiencies in the Virtues.

Benevolence, the Virtue related to the Liver's Psyche, appears to be totally absent, so imbalances in this Organ can be seen in Vine people. Let's remember that benevolence means being capable of including others in the development of one's own life but without detaining the flow of the other person's life; it is about favoring the simultaneous development of both paths. The other person, while fulfilling his own destiny, is a participant in the development of my path. Notice the difference between this way of including others and manipulating for the purpose of taking advantage of others.

Rectitude, associated with the Lung's Psyche, seems to be abolished. The balance between accumulation and elimination has no equilibrium whatsoever; Vine cheats by tipping the scale always to the side of receiving without giving. He lacks the other attribute that the Lung's Psyche confers: being conscious of beauty, of value, of quality. Instead, more importance tends to be placed on maintaining that which is material.

The will to live, associated with the Kidney, is hypertrophied. The Vine person seems to perceive that the only one who ought to live is himself. One of the least recommended things in Daoism is to want more life for oneself and less for others.

Integrity and reciprocity, related to the Spleen, are dissociated. The spotlight is on individual integrity without any reciprocity whatsoever. Vine people (especially primary types*) tend to have a huge Energy reserve because they do not lose it to Emotions and do not exchange it with others.

It is quite possible that deep down in Vine people, and of course imperceptible to them, there exists a deep resentment regarding death.

---

*[Ricardo Orozco, in *Flores de Bach: 38 Descripciones Dinámicas,* proposes two Vine types: a primary type, definable as a sociopath, and a secondary type, which develops as compensation for imbalances in other Flower personality types. —*Trans.*]

I wouldn't say it's fear, due to the relationship that Vine has with Emotions, but more like a need to accumulate body, matter, life, Energy, and control for existing in the world, because without these he would disappear. It is an aspect that deserves further observation and reflection.

Comments

We use Vine Flower Essence to treat piercing pain typical of Blood stagnation and for pain due to Cold that tends to be very severe (for example, in some types of arthrosis).

It's a good idea to keep in mind the people who live with or are around a Vine person; not only might they be terrorized but they may also suffer from Energy deficiencies given that they must develop a great opposing force in order to carry out their life according to their individual path.

The Vine person has the potential to be a great conductor. Conducting really has to do with persuading, awakening enthusiasm. The conductor connects with the necessities of the community in which she lives and knows how to stimulate her society for finding creative solutions. She puts in her part and orients, coordinates, and nucleates a production, which others carry forth, marking the path in concordance with others. It has to do with using power and potential to prepare the ground and to let things happen, to complete themselves.

As far as recognizing one's internal nature and traveling one's life path and purpose, someone settled into a Vine state doesn't have the slightest interest. It would imply an internal perception and listening far from possible in this state. When someone from "outside" has the wisdom and clarity to see what place in the community the Vine person might hold, and the Vine person accepts the task, a qualitative change of great magnitude could occur, and he might begin to walk the path of his destiny.

Wild Oat

Center

This essence has a central role in the system created by Dr. Bach; he himself, in one of his schematic drawings,* put Wild Oat in the center

---

*[See Julian Barnard's *Bach Flower Remedies: Form and Function.* —*Trans.*]

of a circumference whose rays are the other Flowers. Out of Wild Oat, each Flower can be accessed, and each Flower may be seen as a radiation of the essence that occupies center. From the center point it is possible to "see" in every direction.

Center is where agitation stills, where confusion ceases. At the center point, that which is diverse becomes one, and from that unity it is possible to perceive, in a simple and spontaneous way, one's life purpose and the potential one has for bringing it to fruition.

The existential disjunction that this Flower Essence treats is one of the most transcendental, so it is probably valid that it occupy a central place in the schematic drawing. When this dilemma is not taken into account, when it is not even approached, it can become a lighthouse radiating all sorts of dysfunctions and illnesses.

It has never been a simple task to recognize the paths in one's personal destiny, much less dare to walk them. What Dr. Bach has provided us in Wild Oat (not to mention his complete work) is invaluable in this sense, offering us an essence that can help us to come in contact with what Daoists call the celestial mandate.

In Daoism, one of the most noble human efforts is that of connecting with one's celestial mandate and carrying it out, making use of the potentials embedded in each individual's internal nature.* True for both Dr. Bach and in Daoist doctrine, health is closely related to recognizing and honoring one's internal nature and celestial mandate.

While attempts to negate or to modify our internal nature lead to suffering, that which is done in concordance with our internal nature provides joy and satisfaction (Guo Xiang, mentioned in Alexander, "Nutrindo a vitalidade"). So, it is also important not to get oneself mixed up in circumstances and actions that would be contrary to one's internal nature. People in Wild Oat states tend to find themselves in jobs, friendships, or romantic relationships that violate their internal nature.

Human satisfaction and plenitude come from honoring the celestial mandate; Wild Oat helps us come in contact with it. It can do so in

---

*In this context, "internal nature" means the innate state and propensities of the individualized being, previous to its interaction with the world. See Alexander, "Nutrindo a vitalidade."

a way that seems transcendental, helping to clearly illuminate a great portion of our path, or, on other occasions, in ways that seem more humble—like promoting an encounter with some person, or maybe we pick up a photograph from some period of our life, or . . .

Wild Oat Flower Essence promotes the recognition of one's own internal nature; inducing the development of the celestial mandate forms part of therapeutic practice at the Celestial Level of Chinese Medicine.

The Kidney

The Kidney's Psyche bestows us with the will to live—the desire to be alive in a body—which is refreshed and potentized when we get in touch with our life purpose and take action on it. The power to exert will with persistence over time also comes from this Organ's Psyche; it allows us to sustain focus on a purpose, with determination. When, through the light of consciousness, we achieve contact with our life's purpose, the vital potential stored in the Kidneys is transformed into vital force, ready to be used for taking action in the world.

The strength to not get sidetracked comes from Kidney Energy, the root that prevents us from being carried away and tossed around by Wind.

The Liver

The Liver's Psyche has the mission of planning how to develop potentials in concordance with our life's purpose. It is he, *Hun,* who contributes the "how" to do—determining which experiences are most appropriate for deeply living out our celestial mandate. We might say it is he who deploys the strategy so that once life's purpose is identified, it may be carried forth based on concrete events in life. The Liver's Psyche is in charge of finding the true path to walk, in other words, it fulfills an orienting function.

The dissatisfaction generated in Wild Oat situations damages this Organ, promoting a tendency toward stagnation, which could lead to anger, resentment, irritability, cyclothymia (mood swings), intolerance, impatience, bitterness, and depression, among other Emotions.

We might encounter symptoms like hiccups, sighs, a distended feeling in the chest and sides, or the sensation of a lump in the throat, which fluctuates according to the emotional state. Occasionally this may result in a certain difficulty swallowing. Also digestive disorders, menstrual disorders (premenstrual syndrome and others), or breast complaints may be present.

Problems related to instability might be observed: vertigo, tics, tremors, uncoordinated and uncontrolled movements, numbness, paralysis, and others—considered a consequence of the effects of Wind.

The Heart

Thanks to this Organ's Psyche, we are capable of being conscious of ourselves and of carrying out the arduous task of self-awareness. It is Fire that illuminates and through which we might involve ourselves with the depths of Water, where the memory of our celestial mandate is waiting to be activated. Fire, the element that this Organ belongs to, symbolizes the conscience that activates hidden potential in the body. The fruit of the interaction between the Heart's Psyche (Fire) and the Kidney's Psyche (Water) is the power to develop awareness of self, of one's own internal nature, and to bring to our disposal the vital Energy necessary for treading that path.

The Spleen

It is the Spleen Psyche's task to sustain balance between various forces, favoring the stability of the central position. The opposing forces of Water and Fire, and those of Metal and Wood, find cohesion possible through the action of this Organ's Psyche. Thus the forces that rise and fall and that expand and contract are harmonized. Fortify center as the point of reference, and—based on one's personality—one has at one's disposal the opportunity to embody in the world the intentions residing in the Heart.

Another part of the Spleen's Psyche implicates the capacity to memorize. By saying that we must recognize life's purpose, we are declaring that we've already known what it is and need memory to once again identify it in ourselves and realize it.

Comments

As Ricardo mentions, Walnut Essence is more than appropriate for accompanying Wild Oat's action, and likewise Cerato, given that it favors becoming conscious of one's internal nature and acts to fortify center, averting dispersion. The three essences awaken the Kidney's Psyche, so it may provide its qualities of persistence, tenacity, and focused effort.

Ricardo refers to a situation that often presents itself: the path is clear but the task is arduous. Even in these situations, Wild Oat can help us, given that, by recognizing an inner truth, the Heart becomes still and serene, and the simple fact of knowing and beginning to walk in the direction of that truth will begin to provide fruits.

The Flower Essence can assist us in meditation, offering us its help in creating a central place from which we may observe how the mind functions. Consciousness "sees" how thoughts arise once and again, how they stop for a moment and are reborn.

Wild Oat allows us to come out of the periphery, calling us into center. Of the many possible paths and the possible play of various talents, the Flower capacitates us for recognizing what is essential in consonance with our life's purpose, that great organizer of our potentials in action.

Nowadays it is common for children and young people to possess multiple talents, which they might develop with much skill and satisfaction. Wild Oat Essence is useful to them, to help them organize their talents in service to their life's purpose.

When we therapists take the essence, it offers us the service of orienting diagnosis and treatment, making us pay attention to facets that we otherwise would not have noticed and that constitute a valuable and essential orientation.

Regarding disorders related to instability, chaos, and dispersion—in other words, related to Wind—Wild Oat joins the group that includes Cerato, Chestnut Bud, Scleranthus, and Cherry Plum. These can play an important role in the symptoms we mentioned when referring to the Liver.

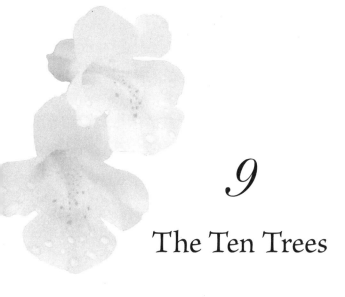

9

The Ten Trees

Cherry Plum

*W*e will begin by situating ourselves in Wood's Movement, in the Liver and its Psyche.

Wood represents expansion—the force that impels movement. If this Energy is manifested in an imbalanced way, we will encounter difficulties in taking action, difficulties getting in gear and expanding our being toward the outlying world, and difficulties in externalizing and saying what we feel and think. Or, we will find ourselves impelled in action, possibly entirely unconsciously or with scarce participation of regulatory mental processes.

These two types of disharmony relate to and weave through each other. When we try to repress all sorts of content—which vary among people—we start betting against the force that lets us spring forth and act. Putting the brakes on that which we would rather keep in the dark (consciously or unconsciously) also damages this expressive force and damages many of our best intuitive, creative, and affective prospects, which we do not control and which we've sometimes not even registered.

Obviously, it is not desirable to have everything internal bud out into action and materialize without mediation. Nor is it desirable that the various mechanisms that sift our actions impose such restrictions that our impulse becomes imprisoned.

Moreover, as Josep states, "a mental impulse, a thought, an idea . . . doesn't necessarily becomes translated into an action or a concrete life occurrence." For this we have moral conscience, exerted by the Heart, which allows us to contain impelling forces, passions, and unconscious contents (all part of the Liver's Psyche), and likewise the constrictive force of the Lung, which puts some healthy, balancing brakes on the Liver's infinite expansive tendency.

Thus we can see that the Cherry Plum state affects these three Organs and that the person who suffers from it feels unable to keep active those controls that the Lung and Heart exert on the Liver's activity. So she decides (many times unconsciously) to make a stronger effort, to put the brakes on more forcefully. This maneuver works for a bit; however, the sustained restriction later generates Liver Energy stagnation, followed by Blood stagnation, and then increased Heat. Result: tension grows and overgrows and finally will blow a fuse, provoking the classic uncontrolled explosiveness.

The Kidney is also implicated given that its balanced activity can prevent the appearance of Cherry Plum states. Kidney deficiency foments Liver excess. Likewise, fear and its family of Emotions are big generators of chaos.

Cherry Plum (also Scleranthus, Cerato, White Chestnut) is very useful in disorders that, in Chinese Medicine, pertain to Wind. This pathogenic factor is a great source of chaos and loss of control.

We see Wind in action when disorders that are presented are missing a fixed location and are changing constantly. We see it not only in uncontrolled movements but also in another facet of lack of control: paralysis.

Wind upsets the direction and situation of things and does so quickly, presenting a panorama of inconsistency and unpredictability.

Common symptoms are spasms, trembling in the extremities, cramps, numbness, loss of sensitivity in some part of the body, vertigo, loss of balance, and repetitive movements like tics.

Some of the disorders that may create a base for the Cherry Plum state are profuse hemorrhages (such as those that occur during birth or heavy menstruation that lasts many days), illnesses that produce high fevers, intense emotional shock or strong Emotions that persist over time, and liquid loss through diarrhea or vomiting.

Staying steady in the Wind requires some strong and deep roots. Jordi tells us that Cherry Plum's roots are shallow and that the Flower provides peace, silence, calm, and equilibrium. We might think that it ought to bury its roots deeper to find wisdom (which lies in the Water element), fortifying the Kidney, but then on the other hand, we may follow the Flower's proposal (the most spiritual aspect of the vegetable kingdom): quieting the mind via various methods, for example through meditation.

As Ricardo mentions, Cherry Plum "helps one accept disturbing or irrational thoughts or images, allowing them to circulate." These thoughts or images may be observed during the meditative practice without the mind becoming alarmed or attached. The Spleen benefits from this practice, given that excess thought affects it. Emotions, which by nature need to move (as Ricardo also mentioned), also benefit. When they stagnate and become repetitive, they generate pathology, harming the functioning of the internal Organs, Blood, and Energy.

Now, let's look again at the Heart, noting that the Heart is Emperor who in the highest court establishes organization, coherency in the personality, harmony, and equilibrium. The Heart's Psyche (Shen, Spirit) is in charge of exercising functions that maintain physical and psychological integrity, that provide the capacity for adaptation to the environment and conscience, and that coordinate and harmonize activity of the Viscera.

When the Heart's functioning declines, we observe disorders occurring in various areas simultaneously. The principal systems of control and communication become disorganized: the nervous system, the neuroendocrine system, the circulatory system. Depending on the degree of lack of control, other systems will join in until the situation reaches such a level of chaos and confusion that the person's integrity is at risk. In these cases the mind loses support and can manifest disorders that could be called insanity, plain and simple.

So it is worthwhile to regulate Emotions affecting the Heart, through the appropriate Flowers, to help it recover its role. Euphoria, excitability, moods that swing between euphoria and depression, sadness, anxiety, and others are Emotions that upset the Heart's capacity to carry out its function as Emperor. Also, we must remember that all Emotions impact the Heart.

Cherry Plum Essence acts on pain. Jordi refers to the hairs on the central vein of the back side of the leaf, telling us about the sensitivity located in the central nervous system.

We have observed that in intense, unbearable pain, the Cherry Plum Essence is very redeeming (see Vohra, *Bach Flower Remedies*); likewise for types of pain that come from cold, that are piercing, or that are due to Blood stagnation, also in distending pain (along with Vine) and those that are erratic and change location (with the help of Cerato and Scleranthus). Elm, as Ricardo mentions, is another essence to consider for accompanying Cherry Plum in treating intense pain. In the Cherry Plum state, pain tends to be generated due to a restriction in the circulation of Blood and Energy and the internal tension that this imposes—tension that struggles to emerge.

Josep's comment regarding the Centaury attitude of some children, oriented around not releasing their power (which could be lethal), reminds me of having noted, in persons with a marked Cherry Plum tendency, difficulties in getting Energy to the extremities and allowing it to manifest itself. This difficulty also carries with it problems in materializing things, a certain awkwardness in fine motor skills, and difficulties controlling Movement.

Untamed Energy that runs amok is draining, reducing energetic resources, often damaging just as much internally as externally.

Tightly maintained contention also leads to loss; that which we retain on one side escapes out the other, and what was lost without our ability to control it was almost always very valuable.

One way to balance Cherry Plum states is to work with the Emotions of the Organs implicated: balance the Liver, fortify the Kidney, care for the Spleen, promote the unexaggerated contention of the Lung and harmony in the Heart.

Regulating the Emotions and Psyches of these Organs—according to each person and always taking into account balancing the Liver—is one way to favor the essence's action.

Elm

Many of the qualities and defects we find in the Elm state are inscribed in Metal's attributes and the Lung's activity. And so, just as impulsive Liver Energy tends to expand outward—at times excessively—the Lung's contracting Energy, when imbalanced, leads to rigidity and introversion.

It is precisely in the area of the Lung where challenges related to spontaneity, perfection, and the Virtues of rectitude and justice are played out. When a person possesses ideals of a certain importance, the delicate issue arises of how to bring them into being without losing one's capacity for adaptation while, at the same time, not allowing their completion to fall to the wayside. It is a characteristically Metal-type balance issue: sustaining structure while still having malleability.

If rigidity is imposed, structure will then drown spontaneity, reducing the capacity to let oneself be shaped by situations but without losing one's own form.

Shielding oneself within a rigid structure may seem appropriate for sustaining ideas, goals, and actions, but it is an adaptation that leads to malnourishment and exhaustion. We know that it ultimately takes a lot of Energy to maintain structure, causing weakness or interruption in achievement.

The tighter and stiffer the structure, the easier it is to overwhelm it. Elasticity affords us more space, letting us expand our limits while maintaining an identity.

Elm Flower Essence favors a balance between rigor and plasticity, giving us back a sense of proportion.

Order, seriousness, schedules, precision, and being methodical pertain to the Lung's territory. They can be qualities applied to daily life, but they can also become defects when exaggerated. The person then becomes strict, dogmatic, obstinate, and perfectionist. The Lung's Energy will become upset, possibly producing symptoms like shallow breathing, coughing, dyspnea, asthma, respiratory mucus disorders, mucus, urinary disorders (like a small urinary reservoir or difficulty urinating), skin afflictions, edema, and others; likewise tiredness and weakness due to a lack of Energy, with reduced immunity.

We are aware of Elm Flower Essence's action on colds. When a person in an Elm state begins to doubt herself and become depressed—added on to her weariness and especially her feeling of being overwhelmed—Defensive Energy is diminished, and so respiratory disorders, including infectious types, survive. When facing external climatic factors, this same debility opens the door to joint problems, with varying degrees of pain and stiffness.

Rectitude, honor, and justice are Virtues belonging to the Lung. It's not all that hard to see how complex it can be to keep balance when exercising such Virtues. One of the most common Emotions that arises as a consequence (as Ricardo mentions) is guilt, inciting Energy stagnation in various parts of the body, such as the chest and pit of the stomach, and affecting the Lung's functioning.

A lack of harmony in the Lung's Psyche creates conditions for obsessive states and a notable fear of whatever might happen in the future, a fear mentioned by Jordi, tied in part to difficulty in cementing ideals and bringing them forth into reality (capacities of the Lung).

In this terrain (the Lung's Psyche), other problematic aspects of the Elm state are at play: the ability to share—in the sense of being able to delegate—and thus transcend one's individualism when carrying out tasks. This would imply less rigidity and self-centeredness regarding how things ought to get done. The Spleen's Virtues of faith and confidence become necessary.

The Elm type tends to be self-assured and acts out of that internal space but loses substance in moments when she feels shadowed by circumstances. She doubts. One way to work with this trait is to develop confidence, not only in herself but also in others, and even more so in the process of life—to have confidence in the flow of the whole. This confidence will not be related to success, failure, responsibility, or perfection; it will relate to the Higher Self, relatively detached from the ego and from personal achievement, though within the field of service to others based on one's vocation.

It could be that Elm folk carry a certain fear of becoming lost in the group, a place in which they may not be able to keep sight of their goals, or a fear that the task cannot be carried out if diluted by group action and thus not conducted by themselves and according to their standards of quality. Flowers that could help in this regard are Water Violet and Gentian.

The relationship between Elm and the Spleen is not limited to faith and confidence. The Flower Essence collaborates with Spleen forces to keep Blood inside its vessels, preventing hemorrhages (Transpersonal Pattern). We have also been using Elm in prolapses (along with Hornbeam). Just as the Elm person's spirits fall from their usual place, his Energy falls and the "level" of his Organs falls; it is the Spleen's task to prevent this from happening.

Digestive capacity is another Spleen-related aspect. Elm is a state of being overwhelmed where there is no room for anything else, making it difficult to assimilate and to learn. We have for a while now been using Elm Essence in this regard, occasionally along with Chestnut Bud and Rock Rose.

We may also use Elm Flower Essence in Dampness disorders. The proper functioning of the Spleen prevents Dampness from accumulating in the body (this may take the shape of mucus, a feeling of heaviness in the body and fullness in the belly and chest, cloudy secretions, dullness, a clogged mind, circulation disorders, edemas). When Dampness accumulates, it generates obstructions and stupefaction of fluid, Energy, and Blood circulation.

Regarding some Emotions and mental states in Elm-type imbalances, we see depression, frustration, and internal pressure (as Ricardo states), which influence the Liver's functioning, fomenting Energy stagnation. The same happens with abatement, an Emotion that creates discouragement and affects the Lung as much as the Liver, reducing the force of vital impulse, draining Energy, and generating stagnation. And finally, the anxiety, worry, and obsession characteristic of Elm states interfere with proper Spleen functioning.

Pine

If we bring our attention to the tree's deep roots, as Jordi notes, we see a relationship between a certain aspect of guilt and a feeling of being too terrestrial, too material.

The Lung's Psyche is the most material aspect of Spirit, the one most related to the body, to substance. When this Psyche is especially strong, there is a great attachment to the body, possibly creating, in some people, an unconscious sense of guilt at the base of their person.

Some people may feel incarnation as a sort of punishment, somehow making them feel unworthy as people. Out of this feeling comes the strong emphasis on perfection, purity, and rectitude, also corresponding to the Lung and Metal; likewise, rigor, which, in Pine's case, is turned against oneself, obscuring one's chance to respond to the environment to make choices in favor of survival.

In making this choice for survival, the mind does not intervene; we might say that the choice is an expression of a survival instinct, a rejection of that which is harmful. In Pine states, this process is violated for the sake of receiving punishment.

Lung disorders will appear as diminished Energy and may be observed as physical and mental weariness along with weakened external defenses of the body: respiratory disorders, mucus, cough, edema, little desire to speak, a weak voice, and trouble breathing when physical effort is made.

Guilt generates Energy stagnation and may also be manifested as a feeling of epigastric, abdominal, and thoracic distension.

Many of the Emotions experienced in Pine states also impact the Lung's functioning, as happens with sorrow, grief, sadness, discouragement, and depression.

The stagnation of Energy seen in Pine states may produce obstructions with circulatory disorders and disconnection between the various parts of the body, mind, and Spirit. In this sense, Crab Apple, Star-of-Bethlehem, and Clematis Flower Essences can be very helpful remedies.

This disconnection also cuts one off from one's environment. Forgiveness restores the connection between people, and dialogue plays a part. People in Pine states imperiously need to reestablish their internal connections in order to maintain a dialogue with themselves.

Ignorance about oneself opens the door to autoimmune diseases. In this same sense we can see how toxic substances, thoughts, and experiences (Crab Apple) accumulate when the door is left open, and the consequences of this negligence.

Accumulation, expressed first as Energy stagnation and followed by stagnation of substances, is related to Pine's mental state of rumination (White Chestnut) and self-involvement, fully impacting the Spleen and influencing digestive processes, cognitive capacity, and learning ability. Corresponding metabolic processes remain incomplete, and waste products continue to accumulate.

The Liver is also implicated where Energy is stagnant, possibly manifesting some of its corresponding Emotions and disturbances. Likewise, the Emotions that a Pine person accumulates can generate internal Heat, resulting in symptoms such as irritability, insomnia, restlessness, a bitter taste in the mouth, and other Heat-related symptoms.

The Pine tree has been associated with longevity, and so it's in our interest to investigate Pine Flower Essence's action at the level of Essence and, as follows, areas related to the Kidney, including congenital diseases. We are also currently evaluating its application in developmental delays.

The union between Heaven (one) and Earth (two) results in the human being (three); the alchemy that transforms that which is terrestrial, converting it into the subtle, occurs within the human being.

We might say that Pine is necessary to move from two (Jordi tells us that it's the most repeated number) to three, and thus to enter into the human dimension.

The human being exists between Heaven and Earth, synthesizing both influences. In Pine states, the person feels these two influences as separate and is unable to incorporate them in the human dimension, which is a place that is perfectible but not perfect. We might say that in a Pine state, the person has lost his sense of place in the cosmos, and so his capacities for relating and participating in solidarity have become injured.

As Mario Satz writes in *El Eje Sereno y la Rueda de las Emociones* (The Still Axis and the Wheel of Emotions): "One who relates, who acts in solidarity, who accepts familiarity as a perfectible fabric, therefore also forgives."

Larch

A person in a Larch state is unable to initiate Movement. What he needs is an impulse strong enough to move him past his conviction of failure.

This impulse must be sought in the Liver and Gallbladder. The force to initiate action and generate projects stems out of the first Organ mentioned. It is about creating Movement—that delicate moment in which inertia is broken. From there, the cycle of Movement has been initiated. This is the first step toward completion.

It is said that character depends on the Liver. Thanks to its Energy, aptitudes of a healthy warrior—a character apt to take risks—may be developed. Here is where we see the Liver's importance in Larch, Mimulus, and Centaury states, for example. We ought to keep an eye on Emotions that affect the Liver, in order to regulate them, and in doing so preserve the Liver's Energy so that it might display the Virtues mentioned above.

Emotional states that lead to inhibition generate Energy stagnation. The Liver is particularly at risk in these cases given that it is one of the Organs responsible for adequate circulation of Blood, Energy, and fluids.

We see how Energy stagnation due to various factors can lead to Larch states, and likewise how an established Larch state can lead to Energy stagnation. A feedback loop is created, making it difficult to recover equilibrium. Energy stagnation, particularly in that of Liver Energy, is the origin of dissatisfaction, frustration, and depression.

Mucus, malnutrition, and trauma (appropriate areas for the Flower's application) are other factors leading to stagnation. These may sometimes explain momentary or chronic Larch states, as can happen, for example, when there is chronic mucus as a consequence of Lung disorders.

Larch Flower Essence favors the circulation of Energy, Blood, and fluids, and we have been using it for this purpose.

Along the same line of what we've said thus far, we may encounter Larch states within symptoms such as migratory pain, distending pain, reiterated sighs, painful and swollen sensations in the chest, sides, groin and lower abdomen, menstrual disorders (irregular menses, premenstrual syndrome with painful swollen breasts, absent menses), the feeling of something stuck in the throat, pessimism, irritability, mood swings, and others.

The Gallbladder, closely related to the Liver, provides us with initiative and courage to realize, to turn a desire into reality. It provides the audacity that a person in a Larch state so badly needs. It is the place of origin for our capacity to make decisions to take on actions favorable to us. It propels dynamism. Through it, we are capable of making judgments. It gives us resistance against psychological pressure in the environment. When the Gallbladder adequately fulfills its functions, we are less vulnerable. As Jordi comments, we can see in the Larch tree's signature its "great sensitivity to the environment."

When the Gallbladder lacks strength, it is difficult to make decisions and to advance. It is very easy instead to become discouraged when facing even the slightest difficulties.

Once an action has been initiated, in order for it to be sustained over time, we need the Kidney's Energy and Psyche. It is he, *Zhi,* who provides the vitality, will, and tenacity needed for carrying out an action without stopping at obstacles, without submitting easily to adversity. All these are truly important attributes for achieving our worldly longings, not to mention following through with transcendental ones. What is more, the Kidney endows us with authority, determination, and self-affirmation.

None of this would be bad for a person in a Larch state; the tree's signature shows us that internally it has Kidney strength but needs more engagement from the Liver and Gallbladder in order to put the Kidney's potential into action.

Although we still need more verification, we have seen various cases of how Larch Essence has helped to fortify the Kidney.

Fear of failure, characteristic of Larch states, drains Kidney Energy and tends to drag the Larch state on and on. Abatement affects the Liver and Lung, easily generating Energy stagnation.

When a person has inherited a weak Gallbladder, Liver, and Kidney, she may be quite predisposed to Larch states.

To paraphrase Ricardo, in Larch states that stem out of Mimulus and Centaury types, we find imbalances in the Gallbladder, Kidney, and Liver. In Larch states that arise out of Scleranthus, we see Gallbladder disorders. In those coming from Cerato, Kidney, and Gallbladder, problems are apparent, and those coming from Gentian show Spleen and Lung problems.

When aggression is used to compensate Larch states, we'll find excessive Liver activity, not absent of Heat, which vastly increases hostility. It is not uncommon to see attitudes that are disqualifying, contemptuous, intolerant, and in constant dispute, seeking self-appreciation through the defeat of someone else. This observation is of course not exhaustive; it is what we have been able to observe up until now.

Let's have a lightning-quick review: thanks to the Liver we generate a project and initiate action; the Gallbladder provides courage and the capacity to be decisive in bringing it to completion; the Kidney sustains action with tenacity based on a sense of authority and internal affirmation; the Heart governs the mind and coordinates the whole process.

Just as in Pine, the Larch state must move from two to three and become conscious that, in the human dimension, the union between Heaven and Earth takes place by doing, especially doing that which leads to fulfilling our life's mission.

Willow

The first Chinese Medicine–oriented uses of Willow were in relation to Dampness. Backing us we had Ricardo's Transpersonal Patterns as well as ancient knowledge about Dampness and the relationships that exist between Emotions found in the Willow state and those of the Liver.

These Emotions disturb Liver functioning, which includes propelling the flow of things in the body, without interruption, in the appropriate directions and at a regular and harmonious rhythm. Thanks to the Liver, Emotions can have stability and the Spirit may be at peace.

Episodes from the past that were experienced as trauma and felt as conflict and that have not dissolved also directly and bluntly affect the above-mentioned function.

Once pent-up anger, frustration, and bitterness destabilize the Liver, it starts to fail at draining water and Dampness; Blood circulation becomes more difficult, tending toward sluggishness and stagnation.

This dysfunction is going to have an influence on digestion and the correct assimilation of food, which will affect the Spleen. And here we find another way through which the Willow state generates Dampness.

So, because digestive processes become difficult, substances that should be assimilated get stuck in a loop, unable to metabolize, and we'll see rumination, generated by Spleen dysfunction, and resentment, an Emotion forged by the Liver and Spleen together. Feeling traumatic occurrences over and over again (resentment) is one way of exercising rumination.

I fully agree with Ricardo when he says that this rumination is the most important mechanism keeping Willow in a state of chronic anger, because Dampness is one factor that best sustains chronicity—and not only with regard to anger but also regarding the whole Willow state.

When Dampness and Heat combine, it becomes more likely for

Holly states to erupt. Heat pushes outward and carries with it anger, which now finally manifests itself. It also affects the skin, as it is through the skin that this externalization tends to happen. A bet is placed between Dampness and Heat, and many times Dampness wins, preventing Heat from externalizing itself. This greatly increases fermentation and likewise refers to the passive-aggressiveness of Willow states.

Incessant return to the causes of disgrace further affects the Spleen, so not only is digestion further hindered but learning is also clouded. The inability to learn is another way that this state becomes chronic. So we can see why resolving a chronic Willow state is not so simple. Some symptoms that may be present are abdominal swelling after meals, weak muscles, weak limbs, weak appetite, weariness, heaviness in the body, little memory, mental weariness, and others.

Dampness is a good terrain for fermentation. It is very much related to that which is hidden and latent. It is sticky and difficult to eliminate, and as such, it continues to generate disorders with symptoms reappearing just like insistent thoughts.

Mental clarity may be seriously diminished as Dampness affects the Heart. Symptoms that may appear include dullness, depression, mental confusion, incoherence, chest pressure, nausea, a full feeling in the epigastric area, and mucus that hinders breathing.

If we add Heat (which is not unusual in the presence of anger and stagnation), we will see intense anxiety, mental acceleration and agitation, much aggressiveness, and insomnia, among other symptoms. Of course not all cases will evolve in this way. This is just one possibility within an advanced and chronic Willow state.

The team for treating Dampness, stagnation, and accumulation is made up of Crab Apple, Chicory, Willow, White Chestnut, Heather, and Chestnut Bud, in the first lineup. Larch, Red Chestnut, and Honeysuckle follow with differing functions. And of course you may find a few others to explore as well.

Finally, a few of the disorders and pathologies that Dampness and imbalances in organic fluids can provoke are mentioned below, not only because we might find them in Willow states but also because Willow Flower Essence can be useful in treating them. This is not an exhaustive list.

. organs: sticky white vaginal discharge

ation: difficult urination, cloudy urine, watery diarrhea or feces, cloudy mucus

- ..... oily skin, skin conditions with thick, dirty-looking secretions
- Joints: limited movement; rheumatic type muscle pain, which can become worse on rainy days; bone deformations may be present; pain due to Dampness is dull, with swelling and occasionally with numbness
- Kidney and Gallbladder: stones
- Subcutaneous nodules (not all of them are related to Willow states)
- Lymph nodes: ganglion swelling
- Thyroid gland: increased volume

Aspen

What you are about to read will certainly not be news to most of us: Aspen is a mystery. It is inapprehensible enough to deserve the Transpersonal Pattern of disembodiment/dissolution. It would seem to be everywhere and nowhere.

Now that we've declared our perplexity, let's look at some facets of this Flower Essence.

According to Jordi, the Aspen tree's roots are superficial, and both Ricardo and Josep agree that a person in an Aspen state is ungrounded. Without exhausting all possibilities, we can speak of three roots in the body: the Kidney, the feet, and Blood. We'll find these three aspects devitalized or as the source of various symptoms, and so should keep them in mind regarding disorders that Aspen people suffer.

Blood is the material base for Spirit, giving it root, allowing Spirit to anchor itself in the body. Without an adequate reservoir of Blood, the Spirit has difficulty establishing itself in the body and tends to float. This may be perceived as a light dizziness or a feeling of floating, even a vague sense of fear, before falling asleep. Some other symptoms may be anxiety, insomnia, a tendency to be easily startled, and periods of accentuated fear and restlessness. We have seen this to be the case in some Aspen states, with varying degrees of intensity, along with a greater or lesser degree of paleness in the face; sometimes the lips may lack a little color or be thoroughly pale. Also, the fingernails may be colorless, dry, and fragile, and the eyes may be dry.

Clematis and Rock Rose people may also present these symptoms. Scarce Blood supply gives material base to these imbalances.

In all three Flower states mentioned, it seems as if the people suffering them were in at least two dimensions at once, like riding between two realities. This is obviously very destructuring. We have noticed that people whose cleft at the tip of their nose is very pronounced, as if it were split in two, suffer from very accentuated Clematis and/or Aspen states; they greatly improve through toning Blood.

Paying attention to nutrition and digestive efficacy and to any possible hemorrhaging (prolonged and abundant menses, for example) can help balance these states more quickly.

The Lung also helps to anchor, making celestial influences earthly. As such, it supports materialization, and therefore could also be affected. What is more, of all the Psyches, its Psyche is the most related to matter and to corporal sensation.

It would seem that this Flower Essence has to do with the process by which Energy, coming out of nonexistence, is materialized and takes shape in the manifest world. Facets of this process, which cannot be decoded or filtered, generate symptoms.

Aspen Essence also intervenes in the inverse process—from matter toward the nonmanifest, when substance tends to disintegrate—by preventing this from happening.

There really is a sense that this essence is connected with that which is nonmanifest, from where changes and situations happening in the manifest world operate.

We are trying out Aspen Essence in any process where regeneration is needed (as the signature shows in the roots' vitality) together with Sweet Chestnut. Also, in everything that precedes our entrance into the world and that has an influence on us (Josep gives the example of Pisces/Neptune) and congenital illnesses (in collaboration with Chestnut Bud and Pine).

We are also trying it as a preventative essence in imbalances that have not yet manifested themselves in the body's functions or tissues.

One application that is very new to my clinical experience is in symptoms and disorders that are rare and that are missing a clear entity, following the idea that these are expressions of things nonmanifest and which in the person are expressed as pathology, as this is the only route of possible expression. This generally occurs both in sensitive, perceptive persons and also in persons whose structure does not give space nor an attentive ear to said manifestations.

Once again, artistic expression provides us with invaluable help for expressing these forces; through this route they find a nonrational means of becoming manifest.

Hornbeam

Increasing one's available Energy supply stabilizes and strengthens the mind. This is why increasing Energy is so helpful in Hornbeam states. One may go about his tasks, facing the less captivating ones or those that are decidedly unpleasant, while still working in the areas where he wishes to create changes.

The Spleen fulfills a prominent role in Energy production. After birth, the Spleen and Stomach form one of the most important resources for the production of Energy, Blood, and organic fluids. Worry, obsession, and too much thinking all disturb the Spleen's functions, among them, Energy production. The same goes for using intellectual capacities during multiple hours without adequate rest.

Sometimes, a little increase in Energy flow improves spirits and physical tone, allowing one to see things with more clarity and providing the necessary strength for change. In some treatments that fail to evolve, especially when the person has a certain clarity about what it is he needs to modify but still can't manage to do so, toning Energy allows him to move past his limitations.

Nostalgia and anxiety, like self-centeredness, also have a negative impact on the Spleen. The great amount of Energy carried away by Emotions and harmful mental states ceases to be available for assimilating, nourishing, and transporting nutrients to the totality of the person. Treating these mental states with their corresponding essences (White Chestnut, Crab Apple, Honeysuckle, to name a few) is one way to help the action of Hornbeam Essence. Gentian for negativity, as Ricardo states, also acts on the Spleen, given that doubt and a lack of faith injure this Organ.

If the Spleen is in balance, it secretes fewer thoughts; the mind becomes still. It is easier to concentrate, to pay attention, to be more in the here and now. We can take the vehicle off autopilot.

Some symptoms that may indicate a need to increase Energy are physical and mental weariness, a feeling of weakness in the extremities, spontaneous perspiration or perspiring under minimal effort, less resistance to changes in the weather, little desire to speak, weak voice, abdominal distension, and others.

The Spleen's activity also helps us to understand some applications of Hornbeam Flower Essence as indicated by the Transpersonal Pattern.* This Organ strengthens and tones the muscles, nourishing them. It influences connective tissues and takes care of nourishing the whole organism. The other Organs depend upon the nourishment it provides. By generating Blood and Energy, it can strengthen any tissue. What is more, this Organ not only produces Blood and Energy, but it also makes sure these get to where they are needed (in the case of temporary weakness) by way of the meridians and blood vessels. Its activity prevents flaccidity and is also related to lymphatic and body fluid circulation.

Hornbeam Essence may also be used to help treat Dampness and stagnation disorders such as mucus, joint pain, edemas, diarrhea, and so on (see Willow).

Dysfunctions caused by Dampness can generate lethargy. The Spirit becomes heavy. Energy tends to drop down a level, and the person loses impetus. Events seem to occur in slow motion. Weariness appears.

Other applications being corroborated have to do with hemorrhages (with the help of Walnut and Elm) and in prolapses.

Finally, let's not forget to take the Lung into consideration as it is another Organ generating Energy, so we might need its help for resolving a Hornbeam state.

Sweet Chestnut

The darkness and profound anguish in which a person experiencing a Sweet Chestnut state may be submerged remind us of the abysmal depths of Water. This enveloping darkness seals off even the most minute speck of light or slightest point of reference that might support the person for reconfiguring the world.

---

*[Hornbeam's Transpersonal Pattern, according to Ricardo Orozco, is lassitude and temporary weakness. See *Flores de Bach: Manual de Aplicaciones Locales* and *Flores de Bach: 38 Descripciones Dinámicas. —Trans.*]

Water is the area where we find the end and the beginning of the life cycle—potential life in a latent state. It isn't just darkness but also silence—the closest thing to emptiness in the manifest world—so it is not surprising that when in contact with this state of being, there comes a sense of finality and of anguish.

We really are quite poorly equipped in modern society for such an intense encounter. Life is so full of things, the mind is so replete with worries, thoughts, and contents of all sorts, that the impact is huge. Such is the magnitude of the experience that ordinary perception is suspended and a breech opens to new potential, new ways of being in the world.

To speak of Water is to speak of the Kidney, which is where ancestral Energy (the Energy we've inherited from our ancestors) inhabits the human being. In Chinese terms, we could call the Kidney the source of "Pre-Heaven Essence."

The first thing we can say about Sweet Chestnut is that this state demands a great deal of Kidney Energy, which is why it is not uncommon that after experiencing this state, a deep weariness overcomes the person. They had to tap their deep Energy reserves. This is how we use Essential Kidney Energy during difficult times and chronic illness, and why it is said that in the case of any chronic illness, or deep or difficult life change, the Kidney needs toning.

A good portion of the symptoms that appear in an acute Sweet Chestnut state correspond with imbalances in the Heart and Kidney, Organs that are affected by overwhelming fear and terror, as Ricardo mentioned. The Lung is also affected in these circumstances. As a consequence, the circulation of Energy becomes disorganized and the direction of its Movements is altered.

This Flower is also related to regeneration, and the Kidney is in charge of the capacity to regenerate. When tissues need repairing, it is the Kidney that gets asked to give up its Energy, specifically for bone tissue, bone marrow, spinal cord and brain tissue, and teeth but also for any other aspect of the body's substance possibly needing regeneration.

Following birth, the Kidney controls the cycles of development and growth, and from what we know about the Sweet Chestnut Flower, we could include the potential for cycles of transformation. Each one of these transformative moments in life is a signpost also constituting a fissure through which other states of being may be accessed—a split that opens up to evolution.

Some of the dysfunctions arising when the ancestral Energy stored in the Kidney is not able to properly fulfill its functions are poor bone development, infertility, repeated miscarriages, tooth deterioration, hair loss, and premature aging. In children, rickets, mental delays, and delays in fontanel closure may occur.

A person's constitution also depends on the Kidney. When this is not robust enough, the following conditions may appear: predisposition to colds, flu, and other external pathogenic factors, chronic rhinitis, allergic rhinitis.

Problems at the mental level may be observed, such as poor concentration, reduced memory, dizziness, a feeling of emptiness in the head. It is also common to experience disruptions in sexual functioning, weakness in the knees, deafness, and tinnitus.

I'm not saying that this myriad of symptoms may be totally resolved by taking Sweet Chestnut Flower Essence; we have, though, observed that it does sometimes bring about great improvement. We use it in conjunction with Olive, and with regard to those aspects related with regeneration, we mix it with Clematis and Aspen.

Another of the Flower Essence's applications is in congenital diseases, in which case it gets accompanied by Pine, Aspen, and Chestnut Bud.

As Ricardo notes, we are still at the stage of investigation and observation to confirm these effects.

Beech

Both Josep and I felt attracted to Dr. Bach's description of Beech: "For those who feel the need to see more goodness and beauty in all that surround them." And I remembered a phrase that the Buddhist master Thich Nhat Hahn wrote in his book *The Sun My Heart,* "Seeing and loving go always together," in reference to the interdependence of all beings, that the life of all beings is one life. When one achieves this vision, one is overcome with compassion. The paragraphs that follow seem at times to be what Dr. Bach wrote about Beech.

Goodness is a Virtue corresponding with Wood and is related

to the Liver. When the Liver's Energy is balanced, the mind is naturally predisposed to fluidly express goodness. Likewise, as we've said before, cultivating this Virtue helps to regulate the Liver's functioning. Let's not forget that we are not only talking about the Organ but also its whole sphere of influence, including its Emotions and its Psyche.

Obviously, when one is unable to experience goodness, softness, and kindness (all attributes of Wood), it is also difficult to recognize their existence in daily life.

The Liver's Psyche is implicated in various aspects related to Beech. It impels us to relate with others, to have a healthy and balanced degree of extroversion. On the contrary, if this Psyche doesn't have a strong enough expression, the Movement will be reversed, and there will be a tendency to turn back into oneself, creating a sentiment of being isolated. The tendency to introversion effectively favors isolation, creating a feeling of disconnection and of separation from other people and living creatures. Goodness, on the other hand, leads us to get out of ourselves and, at the same time, to be more inclusive and to accept others more, including their ways of thinking and living.

When out of balance, the Liver's Psyche generates a rigid mind-set that lacks the flexibility indispensable for putting oneself in the others' shoes, and on the contrary there is a tendency to reject and to feel rejected, once again creating division and isolation. Intolerance, irritation, and rejection are Emotions of the Liver, in consonance with disharmony of its Psyche.

In the body, this may be expressed as joint stiffness, limited range of motion, difficulties in coordination (very evident when it's also necessary to coordinate one's own movements with those of others, such as in team sports), rigid movements, cramps, tight and knotted muscles, and tingling sensations.

Circulation of Blood and fluids may be disturbed. Digestive and hepatobiliary problems, eye trouble, headaches, insomnia, painful menstruation, and other problems may also appear.

Making a fist is a gesture that has to do with the Liver; in many cases it is done quite unconsciously, even while sleeping. It is an indicator worth noting for prescribing Flower Remedies that act on the Liver, including Beech. People in a Beech state may express their irritation and annoyance through this gesture, sometimes also clenching their teeth.

Tension in the chest and arms, like the symptoms mentioned above, could be related to repressing the need to attack physically—to release tension (which could lead to rage and loss of control) through hitting.

Occasionally we've noticed rigidity or even a crick in the neck as a possible response to the desire to look straight ahead only—to not have to see who is in one's company, at one's side.

The Lung's sphere of influence also participates in Beech states as it relates to rigidity and to difficulties in adapting to change. Also, tendencies toward perfectionism and criticism go hand in hand with an exaggerated and partial sense of justice and rectitude, which, if they weren't imbalanced and expressed as defects, would be Virtues of the Lung. Imbalances in the Lung's Psyche can generate interior-directed Movement, increasing self-involvement and egocentrism. Sadness, pessimism, melancholy, and sorrow are Emotions that could stem out of Beech states.

We must also take the Spleen and Earth element into account. First, because imbalances that Beech states create in the Liver are going to affect the Spleen, given that the two Organs closely collaborate. Furthermore, people in a Beech state would do very well to develop Earth element qualities: to be more nourishing, to encourage growth, to pay more attention to those things we have in common, and to be capable of discovering the most subtle and valuable qualities in others. Fostering a balanced Spleen helps to cultivate these qualities.

People in a Beech state also often deal with food in a very selective manner, which, in the long run, ends up deteriorating the Spleen's functioning, favoring food allergies.

We see that in the Beech state it is difficult to incorporate external elements, to transform them, assimilate them, and convert them into part of oneself, and this difficulty deteriorates the digestive process just as much as it does the learning process.

Allergies, commonly seen in this Flower state, have a clear relationship with the Liver and with the Kidney (for example, Beech stemming out of Mimulus) and may be expressed in areas related to the Lung, Spleen, and Stomach.

Crab Apple

Crab Apple Essence clearly has a wide range of applications and acts on many levels.

Let's begin by talking about some of the pathogenic productions that settle in the body and are created by various factors, including the Emotions and Psyche.

We have generally become accustomed to using this essence for cleansing the organism of any of these productions: mucus, for example, or when urine is heavy with waste product. Still, we are not always aware of these substances' possible consequences. Knowing a bit more about this topic, we'll be able to use Crab Apple Essence in situations where we otherwise might not have considered it. Below we will emphasize some of the more unusual signs and symptoms where this essence may be indicated.

Some of said substances originate in disorders in body fluid management, and we'll be able to recognize these either for what they are or through the effects they create.

Some possible disorders are:

- Pain, nodules, abscesses, lymph ganglion disorders
- Paralysis, hemiplegia, epilepsy
- Palpitations, chest pressure
- Vertigo, mental confusion, delirium, maniacal symptoms, loss of consciousness
- Nausea, vomiting, or a full feeling in the pit of the stomach, as if something were stuck there
- Reduced appetite, rumbling in the bowels, abdominal swelling
- Full feeling in the chest and sides; pain when coughing or breathing
- Heavy feeling in the body; pain and numbness in the body
- The tongue may be swollen and/or present a thick coating

The Kidney's, Spleen's, and Lung's Psyches and Emotions may be disturbed. If so, we'll find sadness, grief, abatement, discouragement; nostalgia, anxiety, worry; fear, angst, phobia; and others. (See appendix 1, "Navigation Charts.")

As we've seen in other Flower states, the substances we've been talking about may also be present when the Liver is disturbed. Emotional disorders are one of the main causes of Liver dysfunction.

On the other hand, Blood stagnation may produce accumulations, generating:

- Pain, usually the piercing kind, constant, strong, and possibly increasing at night
- Swelling, generally fixed: either internal or external with a purplish or greenish-yellow color, painful to the touch
- Some hemorrhages, particularly with dark or coagulated Blood, such as during menstruation
- Dry, dark, cracked, and sometimes scaly skin
- Localized tissue decay, for example gangrene
- Purplish or blackish tone to the nails, skin, face, lips, and tongue in some people

Using Crab Apple along with other corresponding essences—through oral or topical application—can be very helpful in the above-mentioned cases.

It is recommendable to use other essences that help mobilize stagnation, such as Chicory, Larch, and Willow.

In general, we can use Crab Apple Essence in any situation where we find thick, cloudy secretions (Dampness), like vaginal discharge, pasty feces, cloudy urine, cloudy mucus, greasy skin, and skin diseases with thick, dirty secretions. Sometimes these secretions will have a foul odor, an indication that may especially call for Crab Apple.

Although we have already talked about this with regard to another Flower, Dampness in Crab Apple states may likewise present joint disorders of the rheumatic type with limited movement and muscle pain. Pain caused by Dampness is dull, with swelling, and sometimes with numbness.

It is not surprising that the secretions mentioned would have characteristics such as dirtiness and foul odor. Crab Apple's mental and emotional state foments these types of discharges.

The Dampness present in many of the disorders mentioned are characteristically dirty, impure, and sticky. Getting rid of it is quite difficult. In the mental plane, these sensations are associated with shame, a feeling of internal corruption, indignity, or impure thoughts.

Fixed or obsessive thoughts are one of the mind's manifestations of this sticky state, as is laziness or even apathy. There may be considerable weariness. The mind is dulled, so of course concentration and memory are reduced.

Among the Organs, the Lung may be affected by thoughts and feelings of dirtiness and impurity; likewise, its dysfunctions can generate them. The person may present thoughts and feelings related to divinity, religion, and guilt: he may be disgusted with the body, perceiving it as blemish to the Spirit and grounds for all sorts of filth or carnality and attachment such that the person defends himself with fear, rejection, and guilt.

We might also find Gallbladder-associated problems given that this Viscera is related with purity—due to the purity of the fluid it stores—and it emulsifies fats.

Both the Lung and Gallbladder are related to justice. If this Virtue is conceptualized out of proportion, it will generate fertile ground for guilt and feelings of impurity and shame.

Crab Apple Flower Essence is of great help for the functioning of all Organs that fulfill secretory functions, such as the Lung, Spleen, Liver, Kidney, skin, Large Intestine, respiratory mucus, and others.

10

The Last Nine

Walnut

$\mathcal{I}$t is no small matter that Walnut Flower Essence averts Blood loss and, in my opinion, the loss of other organic fluids. Fluids (including Blood) give, among other things, flexibility. We know that the capacity for adaptation depends very much on one's flexibility, in every sense of the word. Walnut's work is even more important as it relates to Blood. Blood is the vehicle of Spirit; in a certain sense Blood is an anchor. It is also the material base for mental activity. The role that Blood plays in following one's path with vitality, clarity, and lucidity thus becomes comprehensible. One way to understand some aspects of this Flower's action is to consider the importance of Blood and fluids.

One of the functions of the Spleen is to prevent hemorrhaging—to keep Blood inside its vessels. The Spleen is also implicated in one's capacity for adaptation by providing a notion of *center,* a reference point. We'll expand commentary on these aspects in the next section on Chestnut Bud.

Walnut Essence acts in strengthening the Spleen's functioning by promoting the production of Energy, vitality, and nourishment.

Liquids permit flexibility. Dryness is not a good state for adapting to change.

Part of the ability to adapt to change includes adaptation to climatic changes and to emotional changes in the environment. In this sense, we've been able to observe that Walnut Essence favors the activation of what in Chinese Medicine is known as Defensive Energy.

Walnut Flower Essence may therefore be used when a deficiency in Defensive Energy predisposes one to easily contract colds, flu, and other illnesses related to climatic factors. The same applies to joint pain, with or without inflammation, grouped together under the term *rheumatism*.

With respect to the "emotional climate" that surrounds us, this essence's action is well known for keeping our surroundings from excessively influencing us to the point that we would be knocked off center and off our own path.

Getting centered—cultivating one's sense of center—is important for finding, and persistently pursuing, one's own path in life. Maintaining consonance with our own internal center prevents external influences from pulling us apart in all directions.

The human being must adjust internally to transformations in the environment—both climatic and interpersonal—and if this happens, health happens; on the contrary, illness is an assiduous visitor. A typical saying in Chinese Medicine is that "man and the universe are in reciprocal correspondence."

Change and adaptation require the involvement of the Lung and the Spleen, both of which also provide Energy for the process.

Jordi tells us that the Walnut tree needs to keep away other species that might grow around it in order to follow its own path of development. Here I will revive a topic we mentioned previously—vulnerability. It is not uncommon to see vulnerable people use intense aggression as a way to defend themselves.

How might we find ways of maintaining integrity and faithfulness to self without relegating completely the use of aggressive force or appealing to extreme aggression? Following what we learned from Jordi about Walnut's signature, we might say that taking the essence foments the capacity for knowing when to inhibit and when not to inhibit the actions of others when these actions are directed at oneself and being able to do so from a place of inner fortitude.

The Lung is one of the Organs that provides us with the capacity for adapting to change. The Defensive Energy we mentioned earlier is related to this Organ.

The degree of vulnerability we possess with respect to emotional influences in the environment depends in part upon the condition of the Lung. If this Organ is weak, sensitivity may be acute, and Emotions "in the air" can influence the person to such a degree that they cause physical symptoms such as headaches and digestive disorders.

When we are unable to manage the changes facing us, the Lung may be affected. For example, shortly after the death of a loved one, a person might catch cold, possibly leading to even more severe and chronic problems related to this Organ.

The Kidney bestows us with constancy, will, and the capacity to persist on our own path without becoming sidetracked. These attributes, when in balance, keep us from getting forced off route by the opinions of others. The Kidney also helps us regulate the fear of making mistakes and keeps us from being at the mercy of a lack of clarity regarding our particular task in this world.

On the other hand, an excess of these Virtues turns them into defects, leaving us more or less incapacitated for dealing with changes and for appreciating others' viewpoints, and this includes receiving advice that would illuminate our own path.

To conclude, I'll comment on Traditional Chinese Medicine dietetic therapy.

Eating walnuts fortifies the Kidney and Brain. It is one of the foods that confers longevity when consumed regularly. It nourishes vital Energy, Blood, the Liver, and the Kidney. It lubricates the intestines as much as it does the skin.

Precaution must be taken, and walnuts avoided, if there is serious internal Heat, phlegm with Heat, or formless or liquid stools.

Chestnut Bud

I agree with Ricardo and Josep that the application of Chestnut Bud Flower Essence is universal. Life is plagued with situations for learning and change.

Our learning is so extensive that it occurs with the totality of our entire being: from our internal Organs, our senses, and our cells to our most subtle and immaterial aspects. Every millimeter of ourselves is exposed to change and learning.

The Spleen controls the functions of the Large and Small Intestines. Along with the Stomach, its sidekick, we are in the presence of the most distinguished members of the digestive system. Assimilation, so to speak, is one of the Spleen's specialties.

So, yes, we are speaking of assimilation in a broad sense: that of nutrients, information, Emotions. We could consider this the capacity to elaborate and transform, meaning to take advantage of that which is subtle and light, and to convert food, information, experiences, and so on into part of our being. And likewise, to nourish ourselves with affection, preventing our starvation of experiences and Emotions, making it possible for them to enter deeply into the whole of our being.

Taking care not to repeat the same mistakes implies the capacity to elaborate, extract, and read that which is subtle and to interpret, come to conclusions, and store it all in our memory. This registry of experiences is one of the Spleen's functions. Being distracted, unobservant, and unable to concentrate are disorders related to imbalances in this Organ.

The learning process is very closely related to the digestive process. It entails a constant separation of that which is subtle from that which is dense, implying the capacity to refine and discriminate, so that ultimately what was external comes to form part of oneself; it is integrated, providing nourishment. Digestive functions acting in harmony help us become aware of what is essential for our learning experience: what we need to integrate and what we need to eliminate.

When the above process does not occur, repetitive experiences are created in the attempt to comprehend, to go back for further examination, to relive. Each repetition is one more opportunity to leave aside any unperceptive or indiscriminate clumsiness and to understand within our Emotions, sentiments, intellect, sensations, body.

Regurgitating, or "repeating," food can be a way of expressing that something cannot be elaborated or comprehended—in short, to be assimilated and learned. It is an indicator that points us toward investigating Chestnut Bud and White Chestnut states. This state may also provoke diarrhea (possibly with undigested food), related to low Spleen Energy and to the accelerated way in which the person processes situations. The person doesn't manage to differentiate and take advantage of that which is nourishing and instead expels it. So we can see how favorable it is to unite the actions of Scleranthus, Impatiens, and Chestnut Bud Essences for propelling the learning process as much as the digestive process.

What happens when we are unable to assimilate in the broad sense of the word? Unresolved situations and substances accumulate, and everything becomes sluggish and heavy. The mind gets dense, bulging. The abdomen also bulges and may swell, especially after meals. Substances that could become pathogens are formed: mucus, phlegm, and heavy cloudy fluids. Energy and Blood circulation is obstructed. The state generated predisposes the person to chronic cycles. A circle of eternal repetition is established, and the capacities for comprehension and elaboration are considerably undermined.

Chestnut Bud Flower Essence can put a stop to the situation, notably favoring the Spleen's functioning. This is immensely important given that, on the contrary, one lacks the base for generating vitality and defenses, possibly leading to vulnerability to external influences. And here we find common ground between Chestnut Bud and Walnut.

As we just hinted by referring to Walnut, the Spleen participates in one's capacity to adapt, not only because it "gives" us our center as a point of reference, but also due to its relationship with fluids. The Spleen metabolizes and transports fluids, preventing their accumulation. We've stated earlier that dryness is not conducive to adaptability; nor is an excess of fluids, which makes us too heavy to change, too sticky, slow and attached to our habits. Excess fluids and substances make us idle.

Without assimilation there is no learning. We learn, really, when we integrate into the whole of our being that which we've incorporated and are able to put it into action when the time is ripe. All this becomes important in traumas. If these cannot be comprehended, assimilated, and integrated, they are relived over and over with their full entourage of pain, placing the body and mind in the same space of alarm, stress, and erosion.

All that which is obsessively repeated decreases Spleen Energy, which will then be unavailable for learning and digesting. When there is no learning or assimilation, Energy is considerably reduced. Weariness, weight loss, muscle weakness (even to the point of atrophy), shortness of breath, prolapses, hemorrhages, and anemia may be present.

Chestnut Bud Flower Essence can be utilized for increasing Energy flow and to enrich Blood in quantity and quality.

Even though we have been focusing on various facets of the Spleen, we must remember that all the Organs intervene in the learning process.

As Ricardo mentions, Chestnut Bud fulfills a notable role as integrator. Its use within a formula amalgamates the action of other Flowers, unifying and giving coherency. These sorts of functions are possible in the Earth element's Movement to which the Spleen belongs.

Red Chestnut

Much of what we've been saying regarding the Spleen is applicable to situations where Red Chestnut Flower Essence's action is needed. The Spleen's Psyche, when in balance, provides the capacity to reflect with logic and comprehension (as Jordi mentions) even in difficult situations. This kind of reflection prevents fear from becoming so excessive that it would dominate one's sentiments and actions.

A person in Red Chestnut state needs to cultivate the Virtues of faith and confidence. As these Virtues relate to the Spleen, when they are cultivated, the Organ's functioning truly does improve. So this in itself is very beneficial for treating states related to Chestnut Bud, White Chestnut, Honeysuckle, Holly, Mustard, Gentian, and Gorse— just to name a few where we have most clearly seen benefits.

As Jordi, Ricardo, and Josep have all stated, both the person who frets and worries as well as the person who is the object of these sentiments lose a part of their freedom, making their development, learning, and growth more difficult. In both people we may find disorders related to mucus, phlegm, and viscous substances already mentioned in Chestnut Bud and of which we will speak again in the section on White Chestnut. Said substances are sticky, dense, heavy, obstructive, and slowing. They can cause pain, a feeling of heaviness, difficulty breathing, digestive trouble, and dullness.

In some cases, the internal accumulation of the substances mentioned, as well as the general state of stagnation, which affects Liver Energy, can provoke arterial hypertension.

When consulting with people who were raised by adults with Red Chestnut characteristics, we would do well to observe how these people manifest Kidney- and Liver-related Emotions, Psyches, and body regions. Although these aspects are not mutually exclusive, depending on the child's constitution, one or the other—or both—of these Organs and their spheres of action may be affected.

When the world—even one's own living space—is felt as dangerous, one's Kidney Energy is in a constant state of alert and will tend to become exhausted and even collapse when facing high-stress situations. There will also be an excessive demand on the adrenal glands. We will be facing Olive and Centaury circumstances with deep, old roots.

The Liver may be damaged given that another form of reacting to the world's dangers may be surliness and a warrior-like attitude, in other words, managing fear with the help of anger. In other people, anger arises as a consequence of the persistent restriction on liberty and the frustration that comes along with it.

Kidney deficiency can sustain a Red Chestnut state. Fear is the main Emotion out of which worry and angst arise. As Ricardo mentions, we must keep Mimulus and Chicory in mind, as well as other forms in which fear and angst may be presented.

In a sustained Red Chestnut state, we may find imbalance in the Spleen's Psyche in which it is possible to observe anguish, worry, fear, apprehension, an exaggeration of Emotions and of the situation the person is experiencing, melancholy, digestive disorders, mucus, and localized anguish in the epigastric and abdominal area.

This Flower can be associated with Willow for supporting the elimination of phlegm and mucus. Other essences that are useful for working on disorders in fluid metabolism are Crab Apple, Chicory, White Chestnut, and Heather. Chestnut Bud also collaborates in metabolizing said substances.

White Chestnut

An unmistakable attribute of this Flower Essence is that the mental state it treats directly affects the Spleen. The repetitive, incessant mental activity manifested in White Chestnut states consumes the Energy of said Organ. Or put in other terms, it is the Spleen's Energy that allows for this type of mental activity.

What is more, the mental wear and tear this state produces is a drain on Essential Energy.

When the Spleen's Psyche is disturbed, the mind is inhabited by fixed ideas and numerous worries—decidedly obsessive. Clearly, if the mind is so "full," it doesn't have much space for paying attention to the environment or for carrying out any sort of activity that requires clear and present participation.

And what can we say about one's ability to learn when in this state? Answer: It is seriously compromised!

The result of this kind of energetic erosion may be evident in symptoms like weariness, soft stools, missing appetite, chest and abdominal distension, vertigo, insomnia or disturbed sleep, palpitations, reduced memory, mental asthenia (weakness), and weight loss. We would be wise to talk with our patient about any possible White Chestnut states when facing these disorders.

The digestive process is particularly affected, and as such, one of the sources of Energy production is disturbed. Excessive circular mental process creates Energy stagnation, especially in the midregion of the body.

The person likewise feels stagnant, with a heaviness, a sensation of not being able to move forward. This Energy stagnation later on can create Liver imbalances, giving rise to Emotions like obfuscation, anger, frustration, annoyance, and others.

Another Emotion we may encounter is nostalgia, which sometimes comes along with mental states that affect the Spleen, such as Red Chestnut, Chestnut Bud, and White Chestnut, among others.

Also, having little disposable Energy paves the way for boredom and apathy.

Energy stagnation, along with the hardship to which the Spleen is submitted, can generate phlegm and mucus. As we mentioned in Chestnut Bud, various dense substances begin to accumulate. Due to the very characteristics of an accelerated, repetitive mind, the formation of these substances can happen more quickly in a White Chestnut state.

Once phlegm and mucus are on the scene, the mind becomes more severely dulled. Clarity is further lost, and all this put together—everything we've been talking about—forms a base for this state to become eternal. It is a pathological mechanism that supports the chronicity to which Ricardo and Dr. Vohra refer. Quite often it is difficult to free oneself of these dense substances, which are themselves a petri dish for various pathologies.

The chronicity that the Chestnut Bud state generates, as my colleagues have made very clear, is very much related to difficulties learning the lessons that life offers us. White Chestnut possibly refers more to a mechanism allowing chronicity to settle in and manifest itself.

We mentioned above that Essential Energy may be depleted as a consequence of the situation that the person in a White Chestnut state finds herself. Following birth, the Spleen is the master responsible for nourishing, in every sense of the word. When deficiencies are generated in this Organ, the Energy we acquire thanks to its activity no longer meets basic daily needs. Essential Energy starts coming into play, likewise affecting the Kidney's Energy and functioning. In any chronic situation it is important to observe whatever may be happening in the Kidney and its sphere of action (Psyches, Emotions, body regions, and so on).

In some Lung Psyche imbalances, we'll find obsessive states where the mind fires off thoughts as a way to adapt to life's changes.

Anxiety, which Ricardo mentions regarding this state, impacts the Spleen, Kidney, Lung, Heart, and other Organs. After suffering from anxiety for some time, some of the most characteristic symptoms we might see are dull and pale complexion, dull and pale lips and fingernails, palpitations, insomnia, shortness of breath, lassitude, spontaneous sweating, and little appetite.

It could be in our interest to pay attention to the relationship between states of worry, angst, irritability and anxiety, and blood-sugar levels. Dysglycemia (relatively abrupt changes in blood-sugar levels) tends to be part of the base of these disorders, to such a degree that we would be very wise to regulate the imbalance and thereby support the Flowers' actions. Whole grains fulfill a preponderant role to this effect.

Holly

juiui calls our attention to the thinness of the Holly tree's bark, which is compensated with branches and spikes for protection. This configuration reminds us that one of the routes which vulnerable people can take is that of aggression. Very sensitive individuals—Rock Rose types, for example—who for various reasons are unable to find other ways of feeling safe may protect themselves through aggression.

These individuals construct a perception of the world based on attack and defense, which allows them to hide, even from themselves, their overwhelming sense of fragility.

Regarding the Organs, it is the Liver's responsibility to provide us with a balanced sense of aggression. This Organ's Psyche gives us access to the strength necessary for challenging obstacles, setting boundaries, and facing possible threats. As long as the capacity for externalization that the Liver provides is in balance, we are able to organize day-to-day life and to make plans according to a strategy. Emotions manifest themselves harmoniously. We treat people with kindness. We experience the world as a place of possibility and of communication. We are usually able to maintain a fairly impartial assessment of circumstances, which allows us to make fair decisions with an acceptable sense of proportion.

Under anger's reign, things change.

Anger is not only one of the most destructive, devastating Emotions, it also has a highly disorganizing effect. It bursts forth with brutality and disorder, clearly knocking out any fair and impartial judgment as well as any vestiges of a sense of proportion.

A tendency toward wrathful states notably disturbs the harmonious functioning of the Liver, increasing confusion, disorder, and disorganization. In this emotional landscape, it is almost impossible to stay centered, and the decisions one makes and actions one takes tend to worsen the panorama considerably.

Energy is violently pushed upward in the person when anger takes over, producing an excess in the superior region of the body, evident in symptoms such as vertigo, reddened face, eye disturbances, red eyes, hearing disturbances, and tension in the trapezius and neck muscles. Chances are good that blood pressure increases. If Blood follows Energy, a marked congestion is produced in the head, and the person runs the risk of cerebrovascular accident.

Liver dysfunction clearly predisposes a person to experience anger; he becomes overwhelmed and has trouble keeping himself under control. Balanced, healthy expressions of anger are altered as is the capacity to size up others' intentions. The person develops a tendency to reject and to provoke rejection in others.

Benevolence cannot manifest itself; the Virtue that the Liver bestows is inhibited. This is the Virtue that gives meaning to our self-affirmation in a way that is not damaging to others.

The Spleen (let's not forget that in Traditional Chinese Medicine this includes the pancreas), the Stomach, and digestive functions are clearly disturbed by feelings of anger and annoyance, possibly presenting hiccups, belching, vomiting, diarrhea with undigested food, edema, and swelling.

The Kidney is another Organ affected by anger, manifested as fear, memory loss, and lumbar weakness.

A large portion of Emotions felt during an imbalanced Holly state correspond to the group of Emotions that affect the Liver; likewise, these Emotions arise when the Organ is disturbed.

Holly Flower Essence may be used in the presence of Heat. Ricardo has talked about its ability to act on acute inflammation.

Let's look at a few general indicators of Heat: agitation, redness, thirst, constipation, scanty dark urine, fever, and a subjective sensation of Heat. These disorders improve with coolness. Mucus is yellowish or greenish. There may be dryness. A bitter taste in the mouth indicates that Heat is affecting the Liver.

Notable Heat-related Emotions that may be manifested are irritability, aggression, restlessness (including Agrimony-style physical restlessness), nervousness, and general tension. Cases of intense Heat may also present intense anguish.

Heat can be generated in a negative Holly state, which will affect the Liver and Heart. In the Liver's case, anger, irritability, and aggression will markedly increase. In the Heart, the mind, among other aspects, will be affected, presenting agitation and insomnia and maybe even verbal delirium.

We should note that the Heart is also seriously affected by anger.

Another group of disorders that a prolonged Holly state can provoke include dizziness, vertigo, tremors, convulsions, tics, loss of balance, numbness, and others.

The Liver's Psyche concerns, among other aspects, the capacity to relate with other people. When this aspect is imbalanced, one tends toward isolation and self-enclosure and, as we mentioned earlier, rejecting others and feeling a priori excluded. This state and the Emotions that accompany it set up a situation that is clearly—in Bach's terms—against unity. This is what we might call separateness, an exacerbated sense of discrimination, a loss of awareness of the common origin of all beings.

The problem is that the path of spiritual evolution requires us to practice a sense of community, to travel together. One cannot walk alone. Individualism—any form of feeling isolated—is a path in the wrong direction.

Holly Flower Essence helps the Liver to carry out the difficult balancing act between individuality and belonging to the totality that transcends us.

Honeysuckle

Keeping the past as a point of reference (as Ricardo says about Honeysuckle) is a form of stagnation. All stagnation affects Liver functions, so we can keep all Liver-related aspects in mind when working with people in Honeysuckle states. But the Organ that will be most precisely affected is the Spleen.

Let's start by looking at what happens when nostalgia is a predominant Emotion. This Emotion tends to knot up Energy. The Spleen's Energy becomes blocked, generating digestive disorders. Some common symptoms are weight loss, reduced appetite, swollen abdomen especially after eating, soft stools, and weariness.

A perturbed Spleen Psyche can easily present stagnation of various natures. One of these is an increase in obsessiveness and attachment to past experiences, and when this happens, a great quantity of Energy is tied to memories and is used for evoking them. As we have mentioned on other occasions, the Spleen's Energy is used in digestive processes, in learning, and in assimilating experiences—including those from the past. With the mind focused on the past, a great deal of available Energy is going to station itself there, leaving the digestive process neglected. We could say that the Honeysuckle attitude is, in a broad sense of the word, a form of malnutrition.

Another facet of perturbed Spleen Energy is that things occur more in the mind than in actions in the present moment. So one of the tissues in danger is the muscles because they lose the care and nutrition that the Spleen's functions would normally provide. It is not just a "coincidence" that these tissues are affected; they are also less utilized.

Dry and somewhat pale lips may be an indicator that could lead us to investigate Honeysuckle states, although these signs are not unequivocally related to the Honeysuckle Flower Essence.

A little-known action of this Flower Essence—specified by Ricardo—leads us once again to the Spleen. As we've seen, imbalances in this Organ tie us to the past; exercising memory, especially with regard to that which we've learned, is part of the functioning of the Spleen's Psyche. Surely that which went unresolved and forgotten has still not been transformed into a learning experience, and this is what happens with trauma—as we'll mention in the section on Star-of-Bethlehem—so using Honeysuckle Essence in these situations is of great help.

Fluids can accumulate to form phlegm and mucus as a consequence of stagnation and Spleen-related disturbances. The incomplete metabolism of foods and liquids can give way to denser substances like nodules and cysts.

It is notable that Honeysuckle Flowers rise up at night, as Jordi notes, absorbing the moon and nocturnal influences. It's possible that the Flower Essence has a yin effect; for example, it might act on Heat. I do not have experience in this regard, not having looked from this angle at the Flower's effect. Nevertheless, we might tuck away as a point of reference the use of Japanese Honeysuckle (*Lonicera japonica*) in Chinese pharmacopeia for treating various Heat-related disorders like fever sicknesses, boils, and diarrhea due to toxic Heat.

The Lung, as one of the Organs responsible for adaptation, is also hit by the effects of nostalgia and living in the past. The Lung is often the depository for phlegm, reducing its Energy and therefore its functioning. In older people, the emotional states we've mentioned can be the sustaining factor for Lung-related disorders, often leading to complications that are difficult to treat.

Nostalgia also distresses the Heart; we might see symptoms such as palpitations, disturbed sleep, and varying degrees of difficulty sleeping.

Wild Rose

If we ask where we might find, in the human being, the source of our capacity for struggle and regeneration—which Jordi describes in relation to Wild Rose—we'll get referred to the area of the Kidney.

Kidney Energy, expressed through its Psyche, gives us the will to live. Desires are brought into play, as well as strength and willpower, based on one's sense of having a purpose in life.* The development of one's resources therefore takes on meaning.

In the Wild Rose state, the connection is missing between the strength bestowed to us and our disposition to live—our life's purpose. This is especially important in cases where Energy is not scarce. In order to mobilize Energy, one's life purpose must be clear and full of meaning, and this purpose will serve as a detonator. Even in circumstances where the person does not dispose of a large store of Essential Energy, a strong and defined life purpose confers the capacity to keep moving forward toward accomplishment. Dr. Bach's life is very illustrative in this sense.

When the Kidney's Psyche is weakened through imbalance, the person submits to adversities and life changes without evaluating alternatives or showing any kind of fight. There is a lack of impulse, initiative, and motivation.

A person in a Wild Rose state does not implicate himself in the unfolding of his own life. As Dr. Bach states, he is exposed to all sorts of influences. He does not inhabit himself. He submits to whatever the waves of the environment dictate. With this kind of lack of presence, there is a higher probability of disturbances in immune functioning. External pathogenic factors penetrate more easily.

Rogelio Demarchi says that physical problems can be observed in

---

*The work of Eduardo Alexander is very interesting in this regard; see "Nutrindo a vitalidade."

persons in a Wild Rose state, like ". . . difficulties in elongation and in the joints." These disorders may well be provoked by the invasion of external pathogenic factors like Cold, Dampness, Heat, and so on. Energy stagnation, which may also be present, generates pain. Likewise, disorders in Kidney Energy influence both joint health and immune system efficacy.

It would be worthwhile to investigate the possible presence of parasites and other microorganisms, keeping in mind that there may be infection.

But, what is more, being absent to one's own life may have consequences in the coordination in vital processes. Chaos can ensue. We might keep in mind that the effect of Wild Rose Flower Essence could be helped with Cherry Plum, Scleranthus, Cerato, and Star-of-Bethlehem Essences when facing disorders that implicate various systems simultaneously.

The Liver will also be affected. A Wild Rose state may be a consequence of Liver Psyche imbalances, and it can also generate Liver Psyche imbalances if it persists over time. The Liver's Psyche gives us the capacity to find meaning in life, impulse for action, and the skill to plan one's life based on developing strategies directed toward developing and bringing to fruition one's life purpose. When this capacity is depleted, enthusiasm and desires diminish, projects are missing, and impulse may be minimal. Life's meaning is lost, and there is a very real chance of plunging into depression.

A strong will to live also requires participation from Lung's Psyche, which commands the survival instinct. When this Psyche is upset, the will to live is lost as disinterest gains ground.

In the Wild Rose state, the learning process is interrupted, and there may be afflictions of the digestive system. Weak, missing, and stagnant Energy tends to generate an accumulation of Dampness—as Jordi states—at the digestive level, complicating the assimilation of nutrients and subtle Energy from food, naturally generating deficiencies of Blood and Energy.

Some of the symptoms that may be observed when Energy is lacking are physical and mental asthenia, weak limbs, vertigo, spontaneous transpiration, and susceptibility to coldness and changes in the weather. Also, when Blood is insufficient, the person may present with dry skin and hair, vertigo, palpitations, cramps, insomnia, or pale face, lips, tongue, and nails. Also, it wouldn't be superfluous to observe the Spleen's sphere of influence regarding what we've mentioned in this paragraph.

Wild Rose Flower Essence favors the recovery of Energy. As Josep has stated, Wild Rose, Hornbeam, and Chestnut Bud make a good trio for improving assimilation and toning muscles whose tissue depends upon the Spleen's activity. These three Flowers act on said Organ.

Star-of-Bethlehem

The impact of traumatic events, like all emotional activity, reverberates in the Heart, although the Liver is another habitual target. This Organ is seriously disturbed by conflicts and trauma that have not been worked out and that, remaining unresolved, make their effects felt in the energetic system.

One of the functions of the Liver consists in ensuring the free flow of Energy, thereby maintaining harmony in the functional activity of the Viscera and regulating the Emotions. Just as this function stimulates digestion and assimilation of food, so it does with Emotions and life experiences.

Traumatic events have an influence on this mechanism, generating, on the one hand, what we might call lack of communication between the various regions and substrates of the body and Psyche, and on the other hand, favoring sluggishness and stagnation in the circulation of Blood, organic fluids, and Energy.

It is thought that, that which the traumatic situation provokes gets isolated and stored in some part of the psycho-physical and energetic system with the aim of preventing greater evil. In other words, preventing hierarchically important systems from being affected, such as the nervous system, endocrine system, and circulatory system whose functions of perception, communication, and regulation are of capital importance for sustaining life.

Viewing from another angle, we could say that traumatic events produce a rupture in the person's system of representations, provoking a hole in the person's possibilities for symbolizing. According to psychologist Andrea Rur, the traumatic event can produce the following three effects (among others):

- Disorganization of time-space and/or language
- Uncontrolled repetition of memories or associated sensations
- Forgetting the traumatic event

Looking at the above description, we see that the Liver and Spleen are affected. Repetition clearly indicates that the Spleen's functions of assimilating the most enriching and subtle aspects of an experience, as well as its comprehension, is overwhelmed. As we mentioned previously, Chestnut Bud (along with Star-of-Bethlehem) becomes a fundamental essence when treating the repercussions of traumatic events.

Repetition, a form of stagnation, affects the Liver's capacity to circulate Energy and to regulate Emotions. White Chestnut is another useful essence in these circumstances. Another Flower that is also useful and that acts on areas of the Liver and Spleen is Scleranthus.

Disorganization leaves a person without reference points or direction. So the actions of Scleranthus and Wild Rose Essences are also useful in trauma disorders. Scleranthus Essence also assists in remedying the language disorders that are produced.

With regard to *forgetting,* because the situation could not be assimilated, there is no memory of it. Forgetting is not only a defense mechanism for maintaining a certain amount of psychological and energetic coherency, but also, the event lacks a structure that would allow the memory to operate. It is as if it were something shapeless, unrecognizable. Star-of-Bethlehem Essence acts in these cases, promoting the process of elaboration, granting the person the chance to integrate into the Psyche the Emotions and sensations that, due to their quantity and quality, could not previously be integrated. The Liver, once its functions of circulation and communication are restored, allows the Spleen to carry out the process of assimilation and integration. And as Ricardo mentions, this process does not necessarily happen at a conscious level.

This "unblocking" lets the person recovery the Energy that had been destined toward sustaining the isolation of that which could not be integrated.

This essence's action also promotes the Heart's work in maintaining coherency of the personality and coordination of the Psyche. The traumatic event can behave like an interference field, creating symptoms that have no apparent connection with the traumatic situation and disorganizing the internal Organs' functions and the circulation of Blood and Energy, all of which will impact the Heart. What is more, this Organ allows us to comprehend in a direct way, without the need for discursive processes. Because of this, the Heart is important when it comes time to integrate traumatic events. Jordi also tells us of the Star-of-Bethlehem plant's action at the cardiac level.

Jordi also tells us that the plant contains calcium oxalate crystals, which also make up Kidney and Gallbladder stones. So we could speculate that these types of stones are material manifestations of the accumulation and stagnation of Energy produced as a response to traumatic events.

Yet another look at the plant reveals water and Energy stored in its bulb, reminding us of aspects of the Water Movement (phase)—danger, abyss, things deep and hidden—but also a place of inexhaustible resources, sometimes unknown even to the person herself.

When the traumatic situation is not resolved, it keeps coming back, just as the plant does each year thanks to what it stores in its bulb. Jordi says that during summer, everything unconscious remains below ground as if nothing at all had happened. We could say that in summer, joy and well-being reign. But in autumn, when consciousness and Energy tend to turn inward, when sadness may appear (a new traumatic event or difficult situation could be a trigger), the hidden trauma once again emerges.

The Flower Essence's action provides, as Ricardo states, "mental clarity, vitality, and inner strength," qualities that arise when the Heart's Psyche is strong and balanced.

Finally, I don't want to forget to mention that it is very important to use this essence generously—even when the person appears to have reacted in a balanced and harmonious way to one or various traumatic events—given that the situation can trigger (all too often, unfortunately) severe illnesses like diabetes, Parkinson's disease, multiple sclerosis, and others. The person's constitution and previous state of health will determine, in part, which type of disorder might ensue following the traumatic event.

Mustard

Nowadays, the idea that sadness is associated with the Lung is much more widespread than it was in the past.

Every Emotion provokes determined effects in the human energetic system. Sadness, in this case, affects the Lung and the Heart, generating an exhaustion of Energy, resulting in weakness. Symptoms like dyspnea, quiet voice, cough, and general weakness are among the most characteristic when this happens.

It is also possible to observe abatement of body and Spirit, weak will, lethargy, sighs, thoracic pressure, and crying.

Women may also present menstrual disorders—such as amenorrhea—and Blood insufficiency.

The Lung's Psyche, as we've stated in sections on other Flowers, provides us with the desire to live and the capacity to adapt to change. When imbalanced, the desire to immerse oneself in life is markedly reduced, and instead of flowing effortlessly, the ability to adapt to change requires more and more effort and Energy.

Sadness and grief are two Emotions that considerably take the forefront, occupying a vast area of the emotional landscape. Little by little, disinterest increases. The person also has a high degree of vulnerability.

As balance in the Lung's Psyche further deteriorates, sorrow intensifies and can turn into dark ideas that skirt around death, the highly recognized "dark night of the soul" to which Ricardo refers.

What happens is that, when the Lung's Psyche is disturbed, the capacity to interpret life's losses and gains in a positive light is lost. Part of the darkness and sadness can also be explained because thanks to this Organ's Psyche, we are able to appreciate beauty. When it is weak, everything starts to look ugly and gray. The world loses part of its magic, shine, and color. In the Mustard state, the person suddenly finds herself in the middle of a landscape from some black-and-white Tim Burton film.

Another particularly strong emotional state that may arise is jealousy. And we can relate this circumstance with another aspect regulated by the Lung's Psyche: balance and harmony between the capacity to possess and accumulate, and that of elimination.

Continuing with the Lung, let's not forget that the body's external defenses are commanded by it. When this Organ's Energy and Psyche are affected by sadness, it is no small wonder that there is a reduced capacity to defend oneself against, and adapt to, external pathogenic factors. It follows then that the person is more vulnerable to colds, flu, and other infectious disorders in the respiratory system and of the skin. We know well of the Flower Essence's action in this sense.

This Organ allows us to root ourselves, to inhabit our body and implicate ourselves in life. When this does not occur, many of the symptoms that can be observed in a Mustard state, which we've already mentioned, appear, such as a diminished desire to live and, in depressions, certain corporal insensitivity. The depressed person lacks roots, as if he were absent, disconnected from the present time-space continuum, submerged in himself and his suffering.

It is sometimes possible to observe, in persons who have been under the yoke of sadness for some time, fluid accumulation like edema, many times localized in the upper part of the body.

In the Mustard state it is difficult to sustain the Virtues of faith and confidence, associated with the Spleen, an Organ largely responsible for the genesis of Blood and Energy and which is also indirectly affected by sadness. Thus we can understand why sadness is debilitating. It has a bearing on both of the Organs most influential in the production of Energy after birth (Lung and Spleen).

When the Liver's Psyche is disturbed or loses strength, sadness is one of the Emotions presented, generally accompanied by sighs. The person's capacity to plan her life in accordance with her life's project is lost, possibly turning into depression, diffusing her life's meaning. There is a notable growth in the feeling of isolation, of feeling trapped in the confines of the self. Impulse toward action and expansion is obviously seriously reduced.

Stagnant Liver Energy can provoke alternating periods of sadness. If this Organ is one of the most affected Organs, sadness and depression may be a result of unexpressed Emotions such as anger, resentment, and frustration.

Jordi makes reference to the plant's high sulphur content. This trace element has, among other actions, a purifying effect on the Liver.

Jordi also comments on the plant's pungent flavor. This flavor brings Energy upward and outward and also impels Energy circulation, resolving stagnation. It has a toning and warming action. Notice that the flavor has an action opposite of that which occurs in sadness and depression. When these Emotions have their roots in sentiments like anger, it is wise to use this flavor with caution given that it can generate Heat, increasing and retaining said Emotions. This is not to say that we cannot use the Flower Essence, but it *is* in our interest to keep in mind the relationship between the type of ailment we've been discussing and Flowers like Holly and Willow, as well as Vervain, Water Violet, and Rock Water, with these last three directed toward regulating Heat.

APPENDIX 1

Navigation Charts

I offer these navigation charts as a quick reference for use in the consultation room.

In addition to the material already covered, I've added dreams related to imbalances in each Organ.

Liver

Emotions
Anger. Rage.

Irritability. Contained aggression. Jealousy. Dissatisfaction. Susceptibility. Tension. Impulsiveness. Impatience. Intolerance. Extremism. Nervousness. Depression. Resentment. Frustration. Indignation. Animosity. Bitterness. Repressed anger.

Virtues
Goodness. Benevolence.

Relationships

Movement	Wood
Planet	Jupiter
Cardinal Direction	East
Color	Blue-green

Climate	Wind
Season	Spring
Time of Day	Sunrise
Developmental Stage	Birth, breeding
Organ	Liver
Viscera	Gallbladder
Sensory Organ	Eyes
Sense	Sight
Fluid	Tears
Flavor	Sour
Tissue	Tendons
Manifestation	Fingernails
Expression	Yelling
Emotions	Anger, irritability
Psychic Aspect	Hun
Scent	Rancid
Ways of Reacting	Making a fist
Virtues	Goodness, benevolence
Effort	Ocular abuse

Liver's Physiology

Drainage and Dispersion

Free circulation of Energy, balance of the Energy mechanism, thus harmony in the functional activity of the Viscera. Regulating Emotions. Stimulating digestion and assimilation of food by favoring the Movements of ascension and descent in the Spleen and Stomach. Bile production. Avoids stagnation of Blood, Energy, and body fluids. Regularity of Chong Mai and Ren Mai.

Blood Storage

The Liver retains an amount of Blood to nourish itself and keep its yang under control. Nourishes tendons and eyes. Regulates Chong Mai. Prevents uterine hemorrhaging. Regulates the volume of Blood according to the activity of each part of the body (varies according to degree of physical efforts, Emotions). When at rest, this Blood returns to the Liver.

Liver's Psyche

- Instinctive intelligence
- Astuteness
- Instinct for conservation of the species
- Relations with others, extroversion
- Sexuality: reproductive instinct
- Project generation
- Impulse to initiate action
- Power of the word
- Impulses and passions
- Dreams, desires, richness of the unconscious
- Control of the imagination
- Elaborating strategies
- Finding meaning in life
- Ability to plan one's life
- Important in the creative act

Deficiency

When Liver's Psyche is deficient, things are left unsaid, not externalized. Irritability. Anxiety. Sadness. Sighs. Shyness and fear (insufficient Gallbladder). Intellectual difficulty in organizing daily life. Absence of projects. Inability to elaborate a plan of action for the future. Diminished enthusiasm, impulses, and desires. Feeling of isolation, of recoiling inside oneself. Poor imagination. Depression: loss of the meaning of life. Unresolved traumas and conflicts in the past (greatly perturbing flow and dispersal). Rigidity of thought.

Excess

In excess, interpersonal relationships are complicated in a sense of rejecting and being rejected. Disturbed sleep. Nightmares or dreams of violence. Projects that are incoherent or out of proportion. Uncontrolled impulses. Uncontrolled and excessive imagination.

Angst as Expressed in the Liver

Thoracic-abdominal visceral spasms, episodes of agitation and fury, muscular tension, headaches, sighs. Fear of having something in the head.

Dreams

Dreams of annoyance and anger.

When the Liver Is Deficient

Dreams of trees, forests, walks through the woods, the scent of mushrooms, scent of fresh green plants. In spring, dreaming of being hidden under a tree and not daring to get up. Dreaming of being taken by surprise from behind.

When the Liver Is in Excess

Dreams of being angry, discontent, deceived; fights, rage, judgment.

Gallbladder

Dreams of fights, insults, humiliation, hurting oneself, suicide. Dreams of being inadequately clothed in public or walking barefoot.

Liver: Symptoms in the Body

- Digestive and hepatobiliary problems
- Disorders are erratic and mobile, without regularity
- Migratory pain
- Piercing pain
- Problems in balance, coordination, and locomotion; loss of balance; vertigo
- Accumulation of fluids, edema, mucus
- Hemorrhages
- Eyes: congestion, diminished night vision, blurry vision, dryness, poor eyesight, squinting, crossing, glaring, tearing, myopia, easily contracting infectious conjunctivitis, allergies, yellowish secretions
- Nails: brittle, discolored, lacking shine, dry, soft, deformed; white spots
- Thorax and ribs (hypochondrium): oppression, distension, pain
- Lower abdomen: piercing pain, swelling
- Muscles: lack of flexibility, swelling, diminished sensitivity, spasms, cramps, sensation of the body being hard, convulsions, knotted muscles, trembling, tics, pins and needles, weak tendons
- Headaches, bitter taste in the mouth, feeling of distension in the head, ringing in the ears

- Painful menstruation
- Insomnia, nightmares

Anger, Rage, and Related Emotions as Seen in the Body

Reddened face and eyes. Vertigo. Occasionally, vomiting Blood. If serious, there may be cerebral hemorrhaging, even blackouts. Hiccups, belching, vomiting. Diarrhea with undigested food, edema, swelling. Memory loss, fear, lumbar weakness.

Heart

Emotions
Joy.

Overemotional. Excitable. Alternating euphoria/depression. Sadness. Discouragement. Fury. Anxiety. All Emotions affect the Heart.

Virtues
Courtesy. Correctness.

Relationships

Movement	Fire
Planet	Mars
Cardinal Direction	South
Color	Red
Climate	Heat
Season	Summer
Time of Day	Midday
Developmental Stage	Growth
Organ	Heart
Viscera	Small Intestine
Sensory Organ	Tongue
Sense	Speech
Fluid	Sweat
Flavor	Bitter
Tissues	Arteries, veins
Manifestation	Pulse, complexion

Expression	Laughter
Emotions	Joy, fright
Psychic Aspect	Shen
Scents	Scorched
Ways of Reacting	Suffering, discouragement
Virtues	Courtesy, correctness
Effort	Too much walking

Heart's Physiology

Controls Blood and Blood Vessels

In the Heart, Energy from food is transformed into Blood. It pumps Blood. The condition of the blood vessels depends on the Heart's Qi and its Blood.

Governs Mental and Spiritual Activity

Vitality. Expression of the general coherence of the organism's functioning. Psychological and spiritual aspects. Organizing conscience that expresses itself through the Visceral Spirits. The general harmony of the Viscera depends upon Shen.

Heart's Psyche

- Conscience; coordination of the Psyche
- Perception of our own existence; coherence in the personality
- Conscience of mortality; capacity to contain one's impulses
- Comprehension without having learned
- Memory of past experiences
- Most elevated aspects of intelligence
- Sleep and dreams
- Sexuality: mental pleasure
- Mental clarity
- Serenity
- Clarity of discourse

Deficiency

Depression. Timidity. Alteration of the appropriate perception of situations. Constant complaining. Destructuring of the personality.

Excess
Confusion. Incoherency. Euphoria.

Dreams
Dreams of laughter.

When the Heart Is Deficient
Dreams of fire, flames, fighting against fires, smoke covering a mountain. Dreams of travel. In summer, dreams of being burned.

When the Heart Is in Excess
Dreams of fierce laughter while at the same time feeling angst. Dreams of audacity, of laughing at danger.

Small Intestine
Dreams of crossing great routes, big cities. Dreams of narrow landscapes.

Heart: Symptoms in the Body
- Dysfunctions in regulating body temperature
- Weakness, weariness
- Altered complexion: pale, red, purplish
- Sleep disorders: abundance of dreams, insomnia
- Difficulty with speech
- Thoracic pain and oppression
- Blood deficiency: pale face, palpitations, insomnia, poor memory, vertigo; pale tongue
- Blood stagnation: purplish face, irregular pulse, precordial pain, piercing pain; purplish tongue
- Tongue: stiffness, difficulty speaking, aphasia
- Sweat: abundant or scarce; with the most minimal effort or Emotion; at night; copious and cold

Excitement, Joy, and Related Emotions as Seen in the Body
Palpitations. Alternating between laughing and crying. Insomnia. Poor memory.

Spleen

Emotions
Nostalgia. Worry.
  Reflection. Obsession. Stagnant thought. Anxiety.

Virtues
Confidence. Faith.

Relationships

Movement	Earth
Planet	Saturn
Cardinal Direction	Center
Color	Yellow
Climate	Damp
Season	End of summer
Time of Day	Late afternoon
Developmental Stage	Fullness, ripeness, transformation
Organ	Spleen
Viscera	Stomach
Sensory Organ	Mouth
Sense	Touch
Fluids	Drool, saliva
Flavor	Sweet
Tissues	Muscles, flesh, limbs
Manifestation	Lips
Expression	Song
Emotions	Worry, meditation, anxiety, nostalgia, reflection
Psychic Aspect	Yi
Scents	Fragrant, aromatic, perfumed
Ways of Reacting	Belching, vomiting
Virtues	Confidence, faith
Effort	Abuse of the seated position

Spleen's Physiology

Transport and Transformation
Digestion and metabolism. Extracts the subtle Essence from food and drink, received in the Stomach, and transports them to the whole organism to nourish the tissues.

This function manifests itself in two aspects: in relation to the solid and liquid foods that will construct the base of the Blood, Defensive Energy, and acquired Jing, and in relation to fluids, transporting and transforming Water, and Dampness.

Ascension of That Which Is Pure
The subtle Essence of foods is transported to the Lung. The ascension of the Spleen's Energy sustains the grouping of the Viscera, preventing them from distending and descending.

Production and Control of Blood
It participates in Blood production and as a consequence its function in transformation. It maintains the Blood within the blood vessels.

Spleen's Psyche
- Registration of experiences
- Purpose
- Learning
- Capacity for study
- Capacity to reflect
- Memory of what has been learned, of acquisitions
- Comprehension, memorization, conceptualization, enunciation

Deficiency
Poor memory. Confusion of concepts. Numerous and obsessive worries. Fixed ideas. Shyness. Inferiority complex. Excessive altruism.

Excess
Obsession. Attachment to past experiences. The mind is occupied with experiences and fixed ideas.

Angst as Expressed in the Spleen

Exaggeration. Rumination. Worry. Apprehension. Fear. Melancholy. Epigastric and abdominal angst. Digestive disorders. Phlegm.

Dreams

Dreams about problems. Dreams about immobility.

When the Spleen Is Deficient

Dreams of rocks, abysses. Vast extensions of bogs. Dreams of houses, swept up or destroyed by wind and rain. Tempests. At the end of summer, dreams of building houses.

When the Spleen Is in Excess

Dreams of music and song. Dreams of the body being heavy and unable to move, of wanting to walk or run but not being able.

Spleen: Symptoms in the Body

- Digestive disorders
- Disruption in metabolizing liquids
- Muscular problems
- Dysfunctions related to stagnation
- Epigastric and abdominal pain
- Heavy sensation in mind and body
- Mouth: anomalies in the perception of flavors, pasty mouth, sugary taste
- Saliva: excessive salivation
- Difficulty breathing
- Digestion and assimilation: diminished appetite; distended abdomen, especially after eating; weight loss; thoracic oppression; nausea
- Sensation of pressure on the head
- Feces: soft, pasty, occasionally containing undigested food, chronic diarrhea
- Fluids: mucus, phlegm, edema, dropsy, stagnation
- Deficiencies in Blood and Energy: fainting, vertigo, pale and opaque complexion; tiredness, little desire to speak; easily bruised, spontaneous bruising; blood in the feces or urine
- Muscles: weakness, weight loss, coldness, tired limbs
- Abundant menstrual flow

Nostalgia and Related Emotions as Seen in the Body

Loss of appetite. Distension of thorax and abdomen. Vertigo. Memory deficiency. Insomnia. Restless sleep. Palpitations.

Lung

Emotions
Sadness.

Preoccupation. Dejection. Melancholy. Grief. Sorrow. Anxiety. Restlessness.

Pessimism. Despondency. Angst. Anguish. Discouragement.

Virtues
Justice. Rectitude.

Relationships

Movement	Metal
Planet	Venus
Cardinal Direction	West
Color	White
Climate	Dry
Season	Autumn
Time of Day	Sunset
Developmental Stage	Declination, recollection, harvest
Organ	Lung
Viscera	Large Intestine
Sensory Organ	Nose
Sense	Smell
Fluid	Mucus
Flavor	Pungent
Tissue	Skin
Manifestation	Body hair
Expression	Crying
Emotions	Anguish, sadness, upset
Psychic Aspect	Po

Scent	Scent of animal decomposition, rotten
Ways of Reacting	Cough, expectorate
Virtues	Justice, rectitude
Effort	Abuse of the reclined position

Lung's Physiology

Governs Energy

Breath (respiratory Energy) and Energy throughout the whole body. Captures part of the Energy provided externally by air. Receives the Energy from food metabolized by the Spleen and Stomach.

Thus Zhong Qi is formed (assuring breath and heartbeat). It governs the circulation of Energy, having a very important role in balancing the Movements of ascension and descent, internalization and externalization. It has an influence in the Movement of Blood and body fluids.

Diffusion

Energy, Essence from foods, body fluids. Descends Energy and body fluids (toward the Kidney). Purifies: the Lung's function in elimination.

Waterways

Through its functions of diffusion, descent, and purification, the Lung circulates fluids, along with the Spleen and Kidney.

Lung's Psyche

- Survival instinct, body consciousness
- Introversion, self-centering
- Will to live
- Capacity to adapt to changes in life
- Sexuality: desire, physical pleasure

Deficiency

Due to deeply impacting changes or occurrences in life. Dark thoughts of death and suicide. Thirst for revenge. Desire to leave and abandon everything. Without the will to live. Incapacity to adapt to change. Sadness. Sorrow. Excessive jealousy. Vulnerability. Disinterest.

Excess

Obsessive state. Fear of the future.

Angst as Expressed in the Lung

Sighs, thoracic oppression. Thoughts of suicide. Anguish with sadness.

Dreams

Dreams of crying.

When the Lung Is Deficient

Dreams of white things and forms, metallic objects, marvelous golden objects. Dreams of ghosts. Bloody executions. Dreams of bleeding wounds, dreams of climbing. In autumn, dreams of war.

When the Lung Is in Excess

Dreams of grieving, of being fearful and crying. Flying dreams. Dreams of defecation (Large Intestine). Of large fields, barren landscapes, deserts.

Lung: Symptoms in the Body

- Lung and upper respiratory tract disorders
- Disrupted circulation of fluids
- Skin problems and respiratory mucus problems
- Breathing: cough, asthma, irregular breathing, shallow breathing, shortness of breath, respiratory difficulty, sneezing, snoring
- Poor oxygenation of tissues
- Chest: thoracic oppression
- Skin: rough, dry, the surface of the body is vulnerable to attacks by external pathogenic factors (Wind, Cold, Heat, Dampness, dryness, summer heat), open pores (more sweating)
- Lowered immunity
- Body hair: dry and lackluster
- Fluids: accumulation of phlegm and mucus, edema
- Excessive sweating with minimal effort or absence of sweating
- Little urine, difficulty urinating
- Nose: stuffed-up sinuses, loss of sense of smell, fluttering nostrils, nasal drip

- Throat: pain, dryness, irritation, infections
- Voice: weak, dim, doesn't feel like talking, difficulty speaking
- Energy: asthenia, fatigue, tiredness

Sadness and Depression as Seen in the Body
Shortness of breath, pressure in the chest, weak voice, cough, general weakness. Breathlessness. Laziness, lack of appetite. Palpitations. Muscular spasms and pain in the ribs. Abdominal bloating, weakness in the limbs.

Kidney

Emotions
Fear.
> Apprehension. Phobia. Angst. Cowardice. Panic. Anxiety.

Virtues
Intelligence. Wisdom.

Relationships

Movement	Water
Planet	Mercury
Cardinal Direction	North
Color	Black
Climate	Cold
Season	Winter
Time of Day	Midnight
Developmental Stage	Death, conservation, storage
Organ	Kidney
Viscera	Bladder
Sensory Organ	Ears
Sense	Hearing
Fluid	Dense saliva
Flavor	Salty
Tissues	Bones, teeth
Manifestation	Hair

Expression	Moan, groan
Emotions	Fear, insanity
Psychic Aspect	Zhi
Scent	Putrid, fermented
Ways of Reacting	Trembling, shivering
Virtues	Intelligence, wisdom
Effort	Abuse of the standing position

Kidney's Physiology

Storage

Storage of innate Essence plus the surplus of acquired Essence (Essence from food that was not used to cover the necessities of the organism).

Maturation of sexual functions, fecundity, growth, and development. Production of Blood (bone marrow is an aspect of Essence). Immunity (from Essence).

Generates Marrow and Brain Tissues and Controls the Bones; Governs Water and Liquids

Transports the part that is pure for nourishing tissues. Transforms the turbid part. Evaporation of liquids. Deep part of the body. The Lung regulates fluids in the peripheral parts of the body. The Spleen extracts liquids from foods.

Reception of Energy

Allows for full, harmonious, and effective breathing.

Kidney's Psyche

- Will
- Tenacity
- Memory of daily affairs
- Sexuality: strength, power, and reproductive capacity
- Finish what one starts despite obstacles, without getting sidetracked
- Authority
- Affirmation
- Determination
- Mental capacity to focus on goals and pursue them with determination

Deficiency

Fear. Dread. Indecisive and changeable character. Submits to adversity. Easily discouraged and the mind becomes divorced from goals it set. Anxiety. Angst. Loss of will. Loss of the meaning of life. Extreme apathy. Lack of will and motivation are components of mental depression; toning the Kidney greatly improves symptoms.

Excess

Temerity. Tyranny. Authoritarianism. Obstinacy.

Angst as Expressed in the Kidney

Difficulties in daily affairs. Unable to move forward. Fear, dread, terror.

Dreams

When the Kidney Is Deficient

Dreams of crossing vast extensions of water with feelings of fear and anguish. Dreams of floods and people drowned, of trees and bushes in water or submerged bamboo. Dreams of sailing, of being at the edge of an abyss, of precipices and feeling dizzy.

When the Kidney Is in Excess

Dreaming of being unable to unbuckle a belt, of the spine being broken and not being able to put together the two halves of the body. Separated, the Kidney and back have lost their cohesion.

Kidney: Symptoms in the Body

- Spinal problems
- Growth and developmental disorders
- Problems with fertility, conception, and pregnancy
- Physical debility
- Joint problems
- Vertigo, fainting, amnesia
- Hair: fragile, lackluster, dry, hair loss, early graying
- Teeth: lackluster, dry, stark, cavities, weak, loose, falling out
- Ears: deafness, ringing
- Bones: weakness, fragility, difficulty knitting fractures

- Lumbar area: pain and weakness
- Development: immaturity, regression of genital functioning, sterility, mental and physical retardation in children, premature aging
- Sexuality: impotence, diminished sexual Energy, spermatorrhoea, premature ejaculation, sexual hyperactivity
- Blood: disorders in its production
- Immunity: diminished immune capacity
- Fluids: edema, excessive or diminished urination, frequent urination, dripping after urinating, enuresis, urinary incontinence, difficulty urinating
- Defecation: constipation, early morning diarrhea
- Breathing: breathlessness, asthma, short or shallow breathing
- Uterus: nourishes fetus, deformations
- Menstruation: irregular periods

Fear and Related Emotions as Seen in the Body
- Energy diminished, especially in the Kidney
- Weak and trembling knees
- Incontinence
- Thoracic oppression, trouble breathing, even asthma
- Mental agitation and difficulty sleeping

APPENDIX 2

Ancient Roots

Words of Wisdom

When reading Dr. Bach's work, we might notice that his approach to life, suffering, illness, and healing has deep and ancient roots. This approach implies giving the human being a specific place in the cosmos and therefore also giving a meaning to illness and healing.

Dr. Bach's concept of the human being living life in this world forms part of a long river fed by wisdom from India, from Buddhism, Daoism, Confucianism, Sufism, Kabbalistic concepts, and more—which is to say, his work was fed by profound perceptions whose differences are expressed more in form than in essence according to the era and culture out of which they each arose.

Chinese Medicine has developed over more than two thousand years, nourished mainly by Daoism, whose adherents investigated multiple ways to fortify and promote health, Buddhism, and Confucianism, and this is why we can find among its recommendations for maintaining or recovering health references to spiritual and emotional aspects. Chinese Medicine maintains that one's lifestyle, one's approach to suffering, joy, deception, and ambition, and, of course, the position one takes on the meaning of life are determining factors that influence health and longevity.

The human being is a unity within itself and forms part of a larger unity: nature, which in turn is inscribed within the universe.

Following are some words of wisdom from various ancient sources.

- Insatiable greed and continuous worry deteriorate Essential Energy, moisture, and defenses, so Spirit fades and illness cannot be cured. (*Huang Di Nei Jing*)
- From the point of view of Traditional Chinese Medicine, character is the illustration of one's morality. Only by cultivating one's moral character can one be calm, modest, and peaceful so that the physiological functions can be improved to adapt to external stimulation and resist disease. Without this, the spiritual and physical conditions will decline, and one will easily get ill. (*Sun Zi's Art of War and Health Care*)
- "The Yellow Emperor's Canon of Internal Medicine says, 'A peaceful mind makes one focused and honest, so that the body will not be affected by unhealthy factors.'" (*Sun Zi's Art of War and Health Care*)
- "Only by attaining a lofty realm of thoughts, instead of being swayed by considerations of gain and loss, and being kind and magnanimous, can people live long." (*Sun Zi's Art of War and Health Care*)
- Early detection, diagnosis, and treatment take care of small matters before they become incurable illness (*Sun Zi's Art of War and Health Care*). A change of mood is enough indication for intervention (Howard and Ramsell, *Original Writings of Edward Bach*, "Public Lecture").

The following ideas and suggestions are from chapter 11 of *Sun Zi's Art of War and Health Care*.*

A Serene Heart
- Peaceful Heart, still soul
- Gentle Heart, harmony of sentiments
- Magnanimous Heart, satisfied Spirit
- Pure Heart, clear eyes
- Tired Heart, hard days

---

*[Words were drawn from both the English and Spanish translations of this Chinese text. —*Trans.*]

• Jumpy Heart, trembling flesh

Cultivate serenity as the primary source of health (constant words of an elder).

Serenity Is Acquired: Cultivating High Virtue
• Virtue
• Benevolence
• Justice
• No covetousness
• Indifference; personal disinterest

Enobling Thought, Stabilizing Spirit, and Harmonizing Qi (Energy) and Xue (Blood)
All together these produce . . .

Normal Physiology, Full Spirit, Solid Health
Confucius said: "Great Virtue extends life" (Doctrine of the Mean). He who cultivates Virtue as much as health will get to "be in the paradise of benevolence and longevity."

Being Unworried and Indifferent to Fame and Gain
• If the person is unworried, true Qi flows and Spirit is conserved. This way illness has no point of entry (*Nei Jing*). *Frustrated love, the death of a loved one, failure of a project,* **do not take too seriously,** otherwise, one becomes depressed and will be forever irritable and complaining. In the long run, it shortens life.
• Disinterest of rank and profit, together with tranquillity and contentment, can liven up the Emotions, bring peace to all relations, balance mood, and raise the Spirit. Zang Fu (Organs and Viscera) function in harmony. And mechanisms of Qi maintain their agility. Health.

Exercising Self-Regulation according to Two Principles
• "My life is within me." Maintain constant practice of keeping anger and dismay at bay.
• With a calm, broad mind, conform with that which is.

Serenity in the Heart and Not in the Environment of Life

- Serene Heart: without risks even in complicated situations
- Restless Heart: a person without peace even living out a very pleasant situation

Chart for Pastimes in Old Age and Filial Piety

For a relaxed Heart and pleasant existence:

Five Things

- Sit still.
- Read quietly.
- Contemplate plants, rivers, hills.
- Debate with friends.
- Teach one's children.

Ten Enjoyments

- Study the classics.
- Practice calligraphy.
- Sit with a still Heart.
- Chat with friends.
- Drink a little wine.
- Grow bamboo and other plants.
- Play music and appreciate birds.
- Burn incense and drink tea.
- Climb the rampart or mountains.
- Play chess.

To Pacify the Spirit and Have Good Health

Do not become upset when facing a falling mountain nor a flooding river.

To do this:

- Face reality.
- Love life with a passion.
- Have firm aspirations.
- Behave calmly before any change, reason for joy or for pain.

Following the described methods one may achieve

- Self-regulation
- Stable mood
- Enlivened sentiments
- Getting along with everyone
- A placid Heart
- A clear Mind

Life Is Long

Bibliography

Alexander Amaral de Souza, Eduardo. "Nutrindo a vitalidade: Questões contemporâneas sobre a Racionalidade Médica Chinesa e seu desenvolvimento histórico cultural." Ph.D. diss., Instituto de Medicina Social, Universidade do Estado do Río de Janeiro, 2008.

Arte de la guerra de Sun Zi aplicado a la Conservación de la Salud y el tratamiento de las enfermedades. Beijing: Editorial Nuevo Mundo. 1997.

Bach, Edward. *Collected Writings of Edward Bach.* Hereford, United Kingdom: Flower Remedy Program, 2007.

——. *Heal Thyself.* London: C. W. Daniel, 1996.

——. *The Twelve Healers and Four Helpers.* London: C. W. Daniel, 1933.

Barnard, Julian. *Bach Flower Remedies: Form and Function.* Hereford, United Kingdom: Flower Remedy Program, 2002.

Beinfield, Harriet, and Efrem Korngold. *Between Heaven and Earth: A Guide to Chinese Medicine.* New York: Random House, 1991.

——. *Entre el Cielo y la Tierra: Los Cinco Elementos en la Medicina China.* Translated by Pilar Alba. Barcelona: Los Libros de la Liebre de Marzo, 1999.

Cañellas, Jordi. *Cuaderno Botánico de Flores de Bach: Una guía científica para ver el alma de las plantas a partir de su signatura.* Barcelona: Integral, 2008.

——. *Las Flores de Bach para la Personalidad: Chakras, Principios Cósmicos y Evolución Espiritual.* Barcelona: J. Cañellas, 2010.

Chancellor, Philip. *Illustrated Handbook of the Bach Flower Remedies.* London: C. W. Daniel, 1985.

Cheng, François. *Empty and Full: The Language of Chinese Painting*. Boston: Shambhala, 1994.

Cleary, Thomas, trans. *I Ching: The Book of Change*. Boston: Shambhala, 2006.

Demarchi, Rogelio. *Flores de Bach. Terapia Floral*. Buenos Aires: CS ediciones, 1991.

———. *Flores de Bach: Manual Ilustrado*. Translated by Kato Molinari. Buenos Aires: Lidiun, 1994.

Hoang Ti (Emperador Amarillo). *Nei King (Canon de Medicina); Ling Shu (Canon de Acupuntura)*. Translated by Julio García Lozano. Madrid: La Mil y Una Ediciones, 1982.

Howard, Judy and John Ramsell. *The Original Writings of Edward Bach*. Saffron Walden, United Kingdom: C. W. Daniel, 1990.

Hua-Ching, Ni. *El Tao de la Vida Cotidiana: Una guía para el pleno desarrollo personal*. Translated by Nuria Martí. Barcelona: Oniro, 2010.

Huang Di Nei Jing. Su Wen. 2 vols.: *Primera Parte* and *Segunda Parte*. Madrid: Mandala, 1992.

Kaptchuk, Ted J. *The Web That Has No Weaver: Understanding Chinese Medicine*. New York: Congdon & Weed, 1983.

Levi, Jean. *The Complete Tao Te Ching with the Four Canons of the Yellow Emperor*. Rochester, Vt.: Inner Traditions, 2011.

Li, Ping. *El Gran Libro de la Medicina China*. Barcelona: Martínez Roca, 2002.

Lu, Henry C., trans. *A Complete Translation of The Yellow Emperor's Classic of Internal Medicine and the Difficult Classic*. Vols. 1–5. Vancouver: Academy of Oriental Heritage, 1985.

Maciocia, Giovanni. *The Foundations of Chinese Medicine*. Philadelphia: Churchill Livingstone, 1989.

———. *Los Fundamentos de la Medicina China*. Portugal: Aneid Press, 2001.

Marié, Eric. *Compendio de Medicina China: Fundamentos, teoría y práctica*. Translated by Alfonso Colodrón. Madrid, Spain: Edaf, 1998.

Mariegas, Francesc. *El Tao del Cambio*. Barcelona: L'Entusiasme, 2009.

Nhat Hanh, Thich. *The Sun My Heart*. Translated by Annabel Laity, Anh Huong Nguyen, and Eilin Sand. Berkeley: Parallax Press, 1988.

———. *El Sol, mi Corazón: Interdependencia Universo/Cuerpo*. Translated by Leandro Wolfson. Buenos Aires: Era Naciente, 1993.

Orozco, Ricardo. *El Nuevo Manual del Diagnóstico Diferencial de las Flores de Bach*. Barcelona: El Grano de Mostaza, 2011.

———. *Flores de Bach: Manual de Aplicaciones Locales*. Barcelona: Indigo, 2003.

———. *Flores de Bach: Manual para Terapeutas Avanzadas*. Barcelona: Indigo, 1996.

———. *Flores de Bach: 38 Descripciones Dinámicas*. Barcelona: El Grano de Mostaza, 2010.

Satz, Mario. *El Eje Sereno y la Rueda de las Emociones*. Buenos Aires: Editorial Claridad, 1998.

Sionneau, Phillippe. *Troubles Psychiques en Médecine Chinoise*. Paris: Guy Trédaniel, 2004.

Stern, Claudia. *Remedios Florales de Bach: Tratado Completo para su Uso y Prescripción*. Buenos Aires: Lugar, 1992.

Sun Zi's Art of War and Health Care. Beijing: New World Press, 1997.

Vohra, D. S. *Bach Flower Remedies: A Comprehensive Study*. New Delhi, India: B. Jain Publishers, 2005. First edition published 1992.

Wong, Eva. *Lieh-Tzu: A Taoist Guide to Practical Living*. Boston: Shambhala, 1995.

———. *Lie Tse: Una Guía Taoísta sobre el Arte de Vivir*. Translated by Alfonso Colodrón. Madrid: Edaf, 2005.

Zhufan, Xie, and Liao Jiazhen. *Traditional Chinese Internal Medicine*. Beijing: Foreign Language Press, 1993.

Index